THETA
HEALING®
YOU AND
THE CREATOR

THETA HEALING®

YOU AND THE CREATOR

Deepen Your Connection with
the Energy of Creation

VIANNA STIBAL

CREATOR OF THETAHEALING®

HAY HOUSE

Carlsbad, California • New York City
London • Sydney • New Delhi

Published in the United Kingdom by:
Hay House UK Ltd, The Sixth Floor, Watson House 54 Baker Street, London W11 3JQ
Tel: +44 (0)20 3927 7290; www.hayhouse.co.uk

Published in the United States of America by:
Hay House LLC, PO Box 5100, Carlsbad, CA 92018-5100
Tel: (1) 760 431 7695 or (800) 654 5126 ; www.hayhouse.com

Published in Australia by:
Hay House Australia Publishing Pty Ltd, 18/36 Ralph St, Alexandria NSW 2015
Tel: (61) 2 9669 4299; www.hayhouse.com.au

Published in India by:
Hay House Publishers (India) Pvt Ltd, Muskaan Complex, Plot No.3, B-2,
Vasant Kunj, New Delhi 110 070
Tel: (91) 11 4176 1620; www.hayhouse.co.in

A catalogue record for this book is available from the British Library.

Tradepaper ISBN: 978-1-4019-6066-7
E-book ISBN: 978-1-78817-462-6
Audiobook ISBN: 978-1-78817-556-2

Interior images: Shutterstock

13 12 11 10 9 8 7 6 5 4

Printed in the United States of America

This product uses responsibly sourced papers and/or recycled materials. For more
information, see www.hayhouse.com.

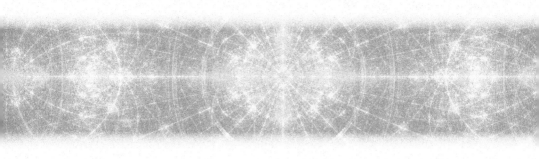

CONTENTS

PREFACE

ThetaHealing® is a philosophy and complete **healing system**, which can be used to change self-limiting beliefs and improve positive beliefs, as well as for self-understanding and evolving spiritually for the benefit of humankind.

These practices are based on the Theta brainwave that I believe creates physical, psychological, and spiritual healing. While in a pure and divine **Theta state** of mind, we can connect with the Creator through focused prayer. The Creator has given us the fascinating knowledge you are about to receive; it has changed my life and the lives of many others.

This book is designed to serve as an in-depth guide to communicating with the **Creator of All That Is**. It is a companion to the books *ThetaHealing*, *Advanced ThetaHealing*, *Digging for Beliefs*, and *Seven Planes of Existence*.

In the first book, *ThetaHealing*, I explain the step-by-step processes of ThetaHealing which are reading, healing, **belief**

work, feeling work, **digging work**, and gene work, and I offer an introduction to the planes of existence, as well as a chapter on children of the rainbow.

The next book, *Advanced ThetaHealing*, provides a more in-depth guide to belief work, digging, as well as deeper insights into the planes of existence and the beliefs that I believe are essential for spiritual evolution.

The follow-on book, *Digging for Beliefs*, defines belief work, and it is necessary to reach an understanding of its contents to fully utilize the practices described herein. In contrast, the *Seven Planes of Existence* book defines the philosophy of ThetaHealing.

It is necessary to reach an understanding of the processes that are given in *ThetaHealing* to fully utilize the practices described in this book. There is also a glossary, which you may find useful if you are new to ThetaHealing.

There is, however, one requirement that is absolute with ThetaHealing and the techniques described in this book: you must have a central belief in an energy that flows through all things. Some might call this the '**Creator of All That Is**,' 'Creator,' 'Creative Force,' or 'the universal intelligence.' With study and practice, anyone can use ThetaHealing; anyone who believes in the Creator or the All That Is essence that flows through all things. ThetaHealing has no religious affiliation.

Neither are its processes specific to any age, sex, race, color, creed, or religion. Anyone open to a belief in the universal intelligence or creative force can access and use the branches of the ThetaHealing tree.

Even though I am sharing this information with you, I don't accept any responsibility for the changes that may occur from its use. The responsibility is yours, a responsibility you assume when you realize that you have the power to change your life, as well as the lives of others.

•••

INTRODUCTION

In ThetaHealing, we believe we can connect with the creative life-force and use our intuition in the most evolved way when in a **Theta state**. When I teach this concept to students, I am constantly asked, 'How do I know I'm connected to the true 'force of the Creator,' this 'life-force of God,' this 'spirit that moves in all things,' or if it is just my own thoughts? How do I know the difference?'

To answer this question, I say, 'You must know yourself. Understand yourself to completely know the difference between your thoughts and divine inspiration.' Generally, however, this ability comes only through experience, so I created a class and this book to help others to know themselves on an intimate level.

ROAD-MAP

ThetaHealing has gone through different stages of development since it began. At first, students learned to go up and 'plug into' the Creator's energy from the Fifth Plane, and in early studies, we found this connection allowed them to reach a Theta wave to achieve results.

Using an electroencephalograph to track brain activity, we found that imagining going up above focusing on the thought form 'Creator' (however the person understood the Creator or God to be), the brain would go into a dream state – a light **Theta brainwave** – and slow to four to seven cycles per second. This seems to suggest that we know, on some level of our being, that there is something to connect to.

Then I taught students to go up past all the planes of existence to the **Seventh Plane** and be in that energy to become part of the pure love of the Creator. This became the 'road-map' to the Creator and was a huge breakthrough. The meditation allowed them to move past the self-limiting dogma in their minds to the realization of an acknowledged connection to All That Is – mind, body, and spirit.

In later studies, I conducted experiments with a more advanced electroencephalograph, which produced computer images of specific brain activity while students were in meditation. All of the electroencephalograph images showed activity coalescing in the upper area of the students' brains. In a similar instance, I measured what happened when a healer was healing another person. Later measurements showed that when in a Theta brainwave, the person receiving the healing is in a Theta brainwave as well. Then both the healer and the subject often go into a Delta brainwave, usually two cycles per second, as the healing takes place.

When I began teaching students to use the Road Map Meditation, my own connection to the Creator was magnified. The next step was to get students to consistently connect to the Seventh Plane and the Creator to understand what might be blocking them from making that connection. To this day, one of the most prevalent questions that students ask is: 'How do I know I am connected to the Seventh Plane and the Creator?'

You are always connected to the Creator, but to come to this realization may take training. The more you imagine what it will feel like, the better the experience will be. Although many people think: *Well, I imagine it, so it's not real...* Think about it. Everything in life has to be imagined before it can become a 'reality.' Don't confuse imagination with fantasy.

I tell students to 'imagine you are going to the Creator.' To help those who think the word 'imagine' means it isn't real, I use the word 'visualize.' Although this word comes with its own challenges, as some say, 'I don't *see* it, I *feel* it.' This is good! I want everyone to feel the energy of being completely loved. So, when you imagine going to the Creator, ask yourself, 'What would it *feel* like to have this experience? What would it *feel* like to have this energy go through my body? What would it *feel* like to be in the energy of creation?'

Here follows the simple yet powerful Road Map Meditation in which you visualize, imagine, and feel the energy coming up from the earth and surging through your body to the top of your head until you feel a light pressure in your crown chakra. This energy goes above your head and travels through the universe, through layers and layers of light.

ROAD MAP MEDITATION

During this meditation practice, it is important to remember 'going up' is a gentle and smooth process. If you are *forcing* the energy as you go up, you may start holding your breath and even get a headache, so remember to breathe normally. You may notice that your tongue is touching the roof of your mouth and begin to belly-breathe during the meditation, both of which are natural.

1. Take a deep breath in and close your eyes. Imagine energy coming up from way deep in the earth, coming up through the soles of your feet, moving all the way through your body, moving up to the top of your head, and making a beautiful ball of light. Pretend you are in that ball of light.

2. Imagine going up past the universe, through layers and layers of light, through a golden light, through a thick jelly-like substance, and into a tingly white light.

3. When you reach this point, say, 'Creator of All That Is, thank you for my life.' Say, 'Thank you, it is done, it is done, it is done.'

4. Feel this tingly white light go through every cell of your body. This is the life-force that creates atoms, the energy that connects us to everything.

5. Take a deep breath in and open your eyes.

Each time you practice this meditation, you will go deeper into a Theta brainwave. The more you go into Theta, the safer you will feel, then your mind will let go, and you will feel the energy.

When I get into this meditative state, I can feel the energy moving all around me, in other people, and in nature. That's because I spend an enormous amount of time working on other people and allowing myself to feel these energies. If you get this deep in Theta when giving healings, it is an amazing feeling. You may feel a rocking energy similar to what happens in cranial sacral therapy when your whole body rocks gently back and forth.

Give your mind a chance to learn how to go this deep in meditation. You naturally go into a deep Theta state when you sleep and are in a dream state, so you will know when you are in this state when you feel as if you are in a dream.

The deeper you are in this brainwave pattern, the more real the experience. You will also find that each chakra opens when you imagine going up to the Creator. Eventually, the chakras won't be separate energy entities but forge together to become one continuous band of energy.

If at any time you feel out of sorts with the meditation, there will be a reason why. It may be due to the beliefs of your ancestors. We inherit many different beliefs, but one thing that makes us who we are is religion. Most of my students come from religious backgrounds, or their grandparents were religious. If their family line was religious, it might be that they have inherited a genetic program that knows there is a Creator.

But if the ancestors in your genetic line believed that everything that happened around them was 'the Creator's fault' in a negative sense, it can make you a little nervous about bonding completely with this energy. But if your ancestors had a different kind of realization – for example, we are a part of everything that is; there is a spirit that moves through all things, that something created life – then the meditation will be much easier for you because it won't be filtered through your ancestors' **belief system**.

This is only one example of how the Road Map Meditation can be affected by the belief systems that pertain to the past, present, and future, and have carried through your life so far. We have energies that make us who we are, and they are called 'belief systems.' What we *believe* is who we are, it is our self-image. When you connect with the life-force that is more than the universe, you are allowed to use this energy, but sometimes belief work is necessary to be able to feel it and believe in it.

I had a student who came to 20 classes but still couldn't visualize anything. She told me, 'All the answers I get are in my mind.' Then one day, it clicked. She changed a belief so she could visualize.

DOWNLOADS

As you connect to the Creator, don't feel that you are as deep into the meditation that you can possibly be. This is where you start doing belief work and use **downloads** that will free your mind. Sometimes it is necessary to download what it feels to be in the Seventh Plane and can make this meditation a better experience. Teaching yourself how it feels, and that it is safe to connect to the Creator, may give you a different experience. Here are some downloads to try:

'I know what it feels like to be in the Seventh Plane with the Creator.'

'I know it is safe to connect with the energy of creation.'

'I am a part of the energy of creation.'

'I have a birthright to be connected to this energy.'

'I am always completely loved and cherished in this energy.'

'Creative energy is the highest intelligence.'

'The Creator loves me.'

'I know what it feels like for the cells of my body to have an awareness of the energy of the Creator.'

Once you have downloaded these **programs**, do the Road Map Meditation again.

Road Map Meditation to Receive Unconditional Love

The second time you use this meditation, it should feel more natural, and you will experience perfect, unconditional love.

1. Take a deep breath in and close your eyes. Imagine energy coming up through your feet. It can start from way deep in the earth coming up through the soles of your feet, moving all the way through your body, moving up to the top of your head, making a beautiful ball of light. Imagine you are in that light.

2.   Go up past the universe, through layers and layers and layers of light, through a golden light, through a thick jelly-like substance into a tingly white, white, white light.

3.   Say, 'Creator of All That is, thank you for my life.'

4.   This time you go on to say, 'Creator, it is requested that I feel the energy of unconditional love in every cell in my body.'

5.   Imagine and witness this energy of tingly white, white light, of perfect love, going through every cell of your body.

6.   Say, 'Thank you, it is done, it is done, it is done.'

7.   Open your eyes.

When you are in the Seventh Plane, remember to permit yourself to feel the energy. I say this because I notice some students stay in their 'ball of light' when they reach the Seventh Plane. But by releasing the ball and turning it into a tingly white light, you will be able to feel the energy of the Seventh Plane. Others go up in their 'ball of light' with their eyes closed, but you need to imagine opening your eyes so you can witness the Seventh Plane.

After using the Road Map Meditation, I believe the brain releases a little more serotonin, endorphins, and maybe growth hormone, in the same way it does during sleep and dream phases.

Also, when you first start using the Road Map Meditation, you may find you crave foods that will replenish the hormones you need to have a better visualization experience. Chocolate, popcorn, organic milk, turkey, and eggs all contain tryptophan and may be helpful. You may also crave avocados or omega 3s, 6s, and 9s, and I have found amino acids to be helpful. This is the mind's response to the meditation asking for nutrition to have a better experience.

RECEIVING MESSAGES

As you learn to 'go up' and hold a Theta state, you will get messages. However, sometimes students describe the messages they receive in readings, and it's clear that they are not from the Creator. The highest energy of love would not give messages the way that some people channel it. The creative energy loves us and is the highest intelligence.

This is because the messages are filtered through the brain and not always clear. Sometimes the healings work perfectly and sometimes they don't. The reason for this becomes apparent if a student feels they need to ask, 'How do I know when I am talking to the Creator?'

It became obvious that I had to take ThetaHealing to a deeper level. To develop their abilities, I had to teach students to:

- Realize that every decision they have ever made matters. In reality, we all create ourselves and what we want to be. If we realized that everything in our lives is teaching us valuable lessons, we wouldn't be as hard on ourselves.

- Trust they were making the right decisions and know why they make them.

- Understand the difference between divine inspiration and the subconscious mind.

- Understand their survival, undercurrent, ego, and higher self.

- Communicate more clearly with the Creator.

- Direct their lives to become more enlightened.

In ThetaHealing, 'enlightened' means being completely aware that you are part of the 'one' energy on all levels of your being. Being aware of other planes and energies does not mean you are enlightened. To be enlightened, you must realize it on all levels together – physically, mentally, and spiritually, not just intellectually.

ThetaHealing is awakening masters to remember that they were once a master of this plane of existence and used the 'one' energy to create. Wake up to the reality that we are all sparks of God and remember how to once again connect to the energy of creation at will.

•••

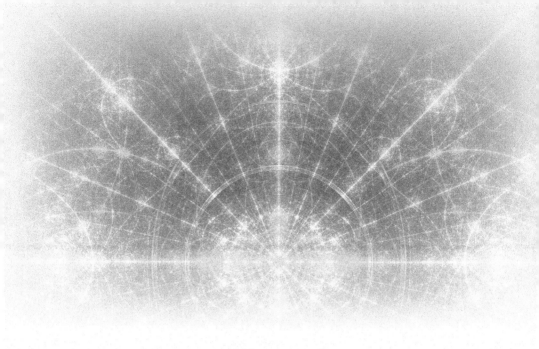

Chapter 1

INSIDE THE
FOUR LEVELS

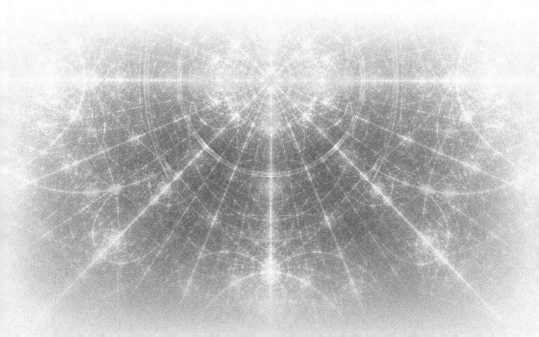

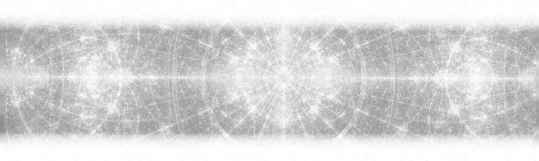

Our spirit resides in our human body. Complete with a supercomputer-like brain, it is the most amazing life support system ever created. This brain learns how to think at higher levels, comprehends the meanings of feelings and emotions and how to control them, and has the job of accessing and processing information.

From the moment you are born until the time that you leave this plane of existence, your brain is accepting information and deciding where to put things. Some of this information becomes beliefs in the mind, and some does not, depending on how important it is to the individual. Our computer brain is constantly shifting and changing beliefs for us to progress.

Very few of us take the time to contemplate just how extraordinary the human mind is and because it is a supercomputer, it never stops solving problems. The mind has two essential components: the **conscious** and the **subconscious**. For these two components to work together, the conscious mind must have an awareness of what the subconscious is doing.

THE CONSCIOUS MIND

The Greek philosopher Plato wrote, 'Perhaps no aspect of mind is more familiar or more puzzling than consciousness and our conscious experience of self and the world,' while in Webster's Dictionary, consciousness is described as 'the state or quality of awareness, or, of being aware of an external object or something within oneself. It has been defined as sentience awareness.'

These definitions are descriptions of the most powerful quality of human experience. All human and animal experiences on this Earth plane begin and end with consciousness. Everything that we have, that we do and feel stems from our awareness. It has created everything physical and is the connection to the spiritual realms.

Even though the conscious mind only runs 10 percent of our brain, it takes external data from our world and makes decisions. It knows when our feelings are hurt and records everything to the subconscious. We need the valuable asset of the conscious mind to direct our judgment calls and must always remember how important it is.

Someone might be listening to a lecture, but at the same time, their heart is beating, they are automatically breathing, their cells are still dividing, along with a host of other processes – all run by the brain without conscious awareness. The conscious mind is like the driver of a car. As we drive the car, most of us don't think about the inner mechanics that make it go, only that it takes us to our destination. Your conscious mind is driving you through your life to reach destination points but may not be fully aware of what is going on with some aspects of the subconscious mind.

THE SUBCONSCIOUS MIND

The subconscious mind runs 90 percent of our lives and is where memories and feelings are accessed. The subconscious is connected to your autonomic nervous system (ANS) that reacts and signals it. In fact, most of your bodily functions are working automatically without messages directly from the conscious mind, which is normal. But how is the subconscious reacting to emotional stimuli and stress?

In this capacity, the subconscious can cause more mischief than you thought possible unless the conscious mind is aware of what it is doing. Most importantly, if we understand how much our subconscious is trying to fix the past, we would be better able to direct our consciousness to the future.

However, the subconscious is not trying to sabotage you. It is trying to protect you by holding on to beliefs and does not discriminate between negative and positive. The subconscious holds the lifetime record of all the earthly experiences and is a virtual storehouse of the beliefs we have accumulated over our lifetimes.

THE FOUR BELIEF PROGRAMS

When a belief becomes accepted as 'real,' it becomes a program and is stored in the subconscious mind. These programs can be for our benefit or detriment – depending on what they are and how we react to them. ThetaHealing teaches that there are **four levels of belief** where we hold belief programs: **core beliefs**, **genetic beliefs**, **history beliefs**, and **soul beliefs**. These levels are used as references for belief work and can be used as a guide for removing and replacing programs in belief-work sessions. Below is a quick review of these four levels. For a more in-depth explanation, you may want to refer to the books *ThetaHealing* and *Digging for Beliefs*.

Core belief level

Core beliefs are like a file of everything that has happened in this life, most of which are learned and accepted from childhood and have become part of us – experiences we have learned something from. These 'beliefs' are held as energy in the frontal lobe of the brain.

Genetic belief level

In this level, programs are carried over from ancestors or added to the genes of this lifetime. These beliefs are energies stored in the DNA that go seven generations back. The genetic level has important information passed down from our ancestors, such as knowledge of virtues, survival, and even from their position in our past, where they are still trying to fix the problems they had in life.

History belief level

This level concerns deep genetic memories more than seven generations in the past, past-life recollections, collective consciousness experiences that we carry into the present, or information from the Akashic records. These energies are held in the auric field of the person of every imprinted life that has ever existed.

Soul belief level

This level is our higher aspect that is always learning. The soul is still learning, so beliefs can be changed on a soul level. These beliefs are generally bottom or key beliefs. Each person radiates a superbly intelligent soul essence. Every part of our soul is connected to us, but our soul is more than three-dimensional because it is a divine spark of the Creator.

●●●

You might find it helpful to visualize the belief system as a tower of blocks. The bottom block is the key, or bottom, belief holding the rest of the beliefs, the root of all the other programs above it. These four levels are a guide to remove and replace belief programs. They are not separate from one another and are supposed to work in harmony. One step deeper into these levels is to know yourself. To know yourself, you have to recognize what you think on a subconscious level. If you know what you are thinking, you will know the motivations of your subconscious mind and how much it influences behavior.

KNOWING THYSELF

Before I started ThetaHealing, I received all kinds of psychic information. But when I did readings professionally, I needed to be focused and accurate. While most of the messages I received about my clients were consistently right, once in a while, they were not. I would torture myself for being wrong, until I asked myself, 'Which voice should I listen to? How do I know what the right voice is? What is the difference between the inner messages from my mind and those that are pure?'

Most people who are intuitive eventually ask themselves these same questions, and this is why it is so important to know yourself. Knowing yourself helps you to know the Creator. Knowing the Creator makes you *limitless*.

Our beliefs are an integral part of us, so when we change beliefs from the past, we make discoveries about ourselves and how a thought form started. One of the greatest things I have discovered in my exploration of ThetaHealing is recognizing the patterns in my subconscious mind and what it is up to.

In turn, this self-understanding has helped me do readings for others. When I do readings, I watch the client's thought patterns. Although similar in each person, every client has a different pattern. The more that I listen to the person speaking, the more I go into their space, the more I recognize their subconscious patterns. These patterns tell me what the client needs to work on. This ability begins by knowing myself with an awareness of my inner aspects of four levels of belief, which we'll explore in the next chapter.

•••

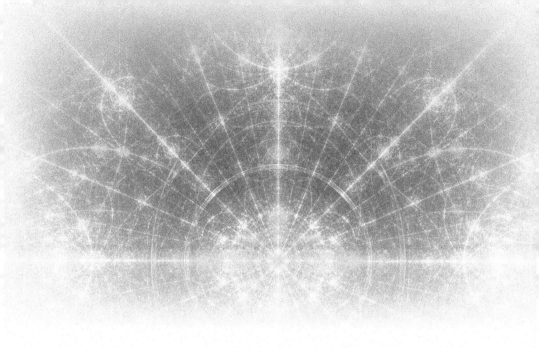

Chapter 2

THE
BELIEF ASPECTS

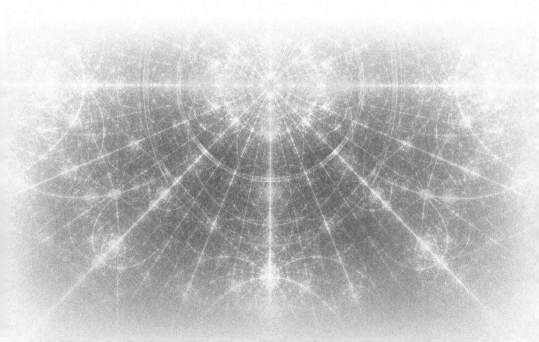

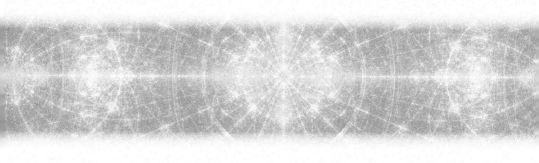

O kay, here's how it works.

Knowing yourself is the realization that within the subconscious, there are **four aspects** associated with each of the four levels. These aspects have a powerful influence on creating behavior patterns, and knowing their motivations is very important for personal growth.

The aspects of the belief system can mean certain beliefs block us from communicating with the Creator. One of them is that when we get a pure message, it has to go through all of the four aspects within each of the four belief levels inside our brain, which I describe in more detail on the following pages. So, we train ourselves to recognize those aspects in others and, more importantly, in ourselves.

As I described earlier in the book, during every class, someone asks, 'How do I know that I am hearing the right answer? How do I know the difference between my own mind and the

Creator?' If someone asks me this, then it is likely that parts of their messages are coming from the aspects of their brain.

When you learn to recognize the four belief levels of ThetaHealing, you begin to realize there are other *aspects* within these levels. The aspects within the levels each have a purpose of their own, and it is important to know if and how they are influencing your communication with the Creator. It is important to know the difference between these aspects and if they are influencing your actions. With just a little effort, you can understand yourself in a much deeper way. This doesn't change how belief work is done. You are still doing belief work on all four belief levels, but with a knowledge of the four aspects.

THE FOUR ASPECTS

There are four aspects within each of the four belief levels.

The core, genetic, and history belief levels share the same aspects and are divided the same way:

1. The survival self-aspect

2. The undercurrent self-aspect

3. The ego self-aspect

4. The higher self and the soul

These first three belief levels have aspects that have a different variation of survival, undercurrent, and ego within them. At the same time, the higher self is one pervasive energy throughout the belief levels. The fourth or soul belief level has aspects, but they have a different energy.

THE FOUR ASPECTS OF THE CORE BELIEF LEVEL

These four aspects are similar to the Random-Access Memory (RAM) – the computer hardware where applications or programs can be easily accessible by the processor. In general, this is similar to the way the survival self operates in the subconscious; it gives easy access to programs that we need at a moment's notice.

1. Core survival self

The core survival self is connected to the memories and feelings of this lifetime. The job of the survival self is to keep us safe and avoid unnecessary pain. Its motivation is to keep us alive and so records pain, stress, and danger for future reference.

2. Core undercurrent self

The core undercurrent self is always trying to figure out and fix what it considers to be problems, no matter what. It is sometimes referred to as the 'shadow self' for those who perceive it as some evil or dark thing. But it can be a force for good or bad and makes no distinctions between the two. Its job is to problem-solve. This self is constantly working on problems, even those that are unresolved from childhood and the past. It is like the undercurrent in the ocean: it can push you up or drag you down. If we are aware of what it is doing, it can help us evolve through self-understanding.

3. Core ego self

The core ego self is how we define, express, and perceive ourselves in the world. Everyone has an ego. However, the ego self (which is neither good nor bad) can be dangerous when it becomes egotism. In some professions, people can get away with egotism, but not in healing. Most healers work with other healers who are unlikely to tolerate someone who is self-absorbed with their own importance. At the same time, some healers mistakenly think they have to destroy their ego to be a healer. This is also going too far because the ego defines us and influences our decision-making, and our decisions affect how we are perceived by others.

4. Higher self

The higher self is above all the other aspects and dedicated to the mission of the soul's evolution. The higher self is attempting to learn as many virtues as possible by creating experiences that develop them and very is focused on completing its **divine timing**. The higher self is a divine part of you too. The more beliefs that you shift and change the more virtuous life you lead, the clearer you become in your decisions, and the more the different parts of your brain develop. The higher aspect of our self keeps us connected to our soul. The higher self is totally connected to the soul, our Fifth Plane self, every belief level, and all their aspects. This aspect is also connected to the other dimensions, which we'll explore later in the book.

When you 'go up' to communicate with the Creator, you may sometimes confuse the higher self with the Creator. It is important to know the difference. The more belief work you do, the more and more aware of your higher self you will become. The higher self is your kindest, most loving part, so make it a goal in life to bring more of it into your everyday life.

Without consciously knowing it, everyone has a continual conversation going on in their head with the aspects of the self. It may be that the higher self is the best voice of reason, and I am not suggesting that you don't listen to them, only that you become aware of their influences.

THE FOUR ASPECTS OF THE GENETIC LEVEL

These four aspects are similar to the software or set of instructions to run your life. Just as system software organizes the activities and functions of hardware, these aspects retain instinctual programs and process ancestral issues.

1. Genetic survival self

This aspect is the instinctual DNA software in the subconscious, which is a combination of survival programs from the memories and feelings of our ancestors.

2. Genetic undercurrent

This is the part of the brain that solves problems with the ancestral family line. These may be issues due to past stress or having depressed-type motivations from ancestors who were poor and desperate. This process is an attempt to solve anything that your ancestors left unfinished. Remember, many of the energies that were sent down from our ancestors are positive.

3. Genetic ego

This aspect has programs that can be good or not so good. Your ancestors might have passed down the program to be proud of your ethnicity or race. But your genetic ego might have the belief that your ethnic background is the 'chosen people' or 'superior people,' which may cause unneeded prejudice.

4. Genetic higher self

This aspect is the same higher self that expands through the aspects of the genetic level.

•••

In ThetaHealing classes, everyone is taught to go up to the energy of the Creator of All That Is. But some people have hidden genetic programs that only become obvious after someone learns about the All That Is energy.

For example, I remember receiving a letter from one of my students saying, 'Thank you, Vianna, for all that you have taught me, but I have found something better. I have found that I can connect to the energy of All That Is.'

I realized that for some obscure reason, she hadn't discovered how to connect to the All That Is energy while studying with me. Obviously, she had only 'gone up' to one level on the Fifth Plane. It was probably weeks or months after the class that she learned about the All That Is essence, so somehow, she hadn't heard what I taught her in class and thought she came up with it on her own. This seems to be common with people who have genetic issues in one of the three aspects of survival, undercurrent, or ego.

THE FOUR ASPECTS OF THE HISTORY LEVEL

These aspects are like a computer network, an internal 'intranet' that processes information from group consciousness and past-life memories.

1. History survival self

This aspect is the group consciousness, past-life memories, and feelings as they relate to survival.

2. History undercurrent self

This aspect is always attempting to fix problems that are associated with something in the history level. It may be something from another life, unfinished business from ancient ancestors, or from group consciousness that the undercurrent is working to change in this reality. Remember, experiences with past lives do not necessarily mean they are all yours.

3. History ego self

This aspect is the ego of all past-life memories, whether they are yours or from an ancient ancestor. It is possible to connect to the ego memories of others and mistake them as your own. Sometimes people realize that they have done amazing things and been powerful people in past lives. Then they act as if they are still Indian chiefs, the Queen of Sheba, Cleopatra, masters or gods, and goddesses of some kind. When this happens, the ego of these past lives can stop them from spiritual development. Remember, everything that has ever lived has impressions, memories in every grain of sand, and drop of water.

4. History of higher self

This aspect is the sum of all past-life memories and other people's consciousness. It is the same higher self that is shared by the other aspects of the history level.

THE SOUL LEVEL

The soul level is the computer processor, hard drive, and power source for life, which receives and processes the combined data to generate results. It is the sum of all the levels and aspects. The soul runs the big picture and is learning from the higher aspect of the self.

Your brain keeps track of every second, every minute of the day with the inner realization that your life experience has a purpose. What is leading this parade is your higher self. It is learning everything it needs for the soul to grow.

When doing belief work, I ask, 'What virtue did you learn from this?' This question is directed to the higher-self aspect connected to the soul. The soul advances only when virtues are mastered, and vices are recognized, confronted, and no longer needed for our advancement in this dualistic world.

Growing through all our experiences, the soul is eternal, yet is still fragile enough to be affected by the harshness of being in a human body. The soul and the spirit are two parts of the same thing. While the soul is multidimensional in nature, the spirit is the ATP energy in the body. ATP, or Adenosine triphosphate, is created by rod-shaped cell organelles that act as power generators called mitochondria. Mitochondria convert oxygen and nutrients into the pure energy of ATP that is used by the cells to function. The electrical pulses of ATP energy are the home of the spirit.

The first aspect of the soul

This aspect is the sum configuration of all the other levels in the third dimension, which includes the Earth and the body that is the house of the soul.

The second aspect of the soul

This aspect is the sum of all the experiences of the soul on all dimensions. There are hundreds of dimensions, and we understand only three. We are so much more complicated than we think.

The third aspect of the soul

This aspect is the best of the ego aspects of all the dimensions. Its nature depends on the age of the soul, whether it is a young spirit or older master, and how old it is in the way of lifetimes. If someone is a young soul, it may be they have an undeveloped ego and are holding on to past anger. But we can only get out of the Fourth Plane when we realize that we have to love others.

An old soul who has graduated from the Third Plane is not going to have a weird ego. If someone is an old soul who comes from the higher levels of the Fifth Plane, then their soul ego is an amazing, beautiful thing.

The soul level rarely experiences egotism. Egotism comes from the lower levels of the Fifth Plane, as baby spirits try to figure out their place in the universe. A genuine ascended master never becomes egotistical on the soul level because they have mastered all the virtues and are totally connected to the fulfillment of others.

The fourth aspect of the soul

This aspect is the complete ascended part of yourself – how far you have developed on all the planes of existence. Once we have learned all that we can from this life, we are left with an ascended self that is amazing.

●●●

Once the first three levels of belief – core, genetic, and history (and the aspects within them) – are mastered in any lifetime, the soul is allowed to advance and evolve through the levels of the Fifth Plane.

The conscious mind is the part of the brain that sorts everything out, so it's important to be fully aware of each of the energies within the survival self, the undercurrent, the ego, and the higher self. This is especially important for avoiding confusion when going up to the Creator. We use the conscious mind to redirect these aspects and create the reality we want in a lifestyle that is comfortable while still fulfilling our soul purpose.

Properly directed, the subconscious and higher self are designed to create experiences as opportunities to learn virtues. When virtues are obtained, new abilities develop and our thoughts become lite, thus making it possible to bend the universal laws. Every experience has something good that comes out of it. On a soul level, we are always learning virtues.

Ask yourself, 'What virtues have I learned?'

•••

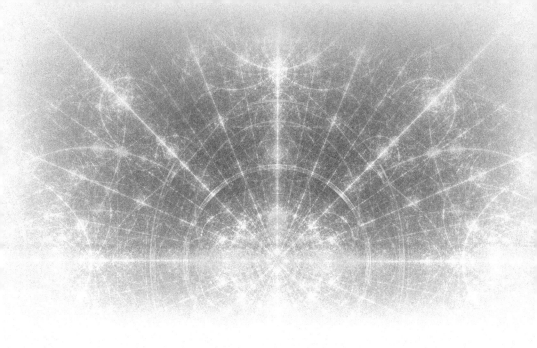

Chapter 3

WORKING WITH
THE ASPECTS

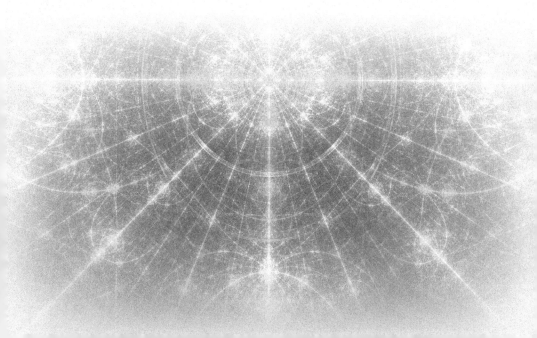

In this chapter, we will explore the aspects in more depth and how we can work with them as healers when doing belief work.

1. THE SURVIVAL SELF

The job of the survival self is to survive no matter what and is an important aspect of who we are. The survival self has many positive attributes. For instance, it holds on to some belief systems, so we don't manifest too fast, because once manifested, we are going to live in what we have created. The survival self wants to protect us from stress. If the survival self is stressed, the undercurrent tries to fix the situation, and vice versa.

The survival self is one of the more obvious aspects of core belief work. Most of the time, when we do belief work, we trigger the survival self. For instance, the program of 'love hurts' might develop in childhood if your mother hit you and said, 'I'm doing this because I love you.' The reaction of the survival self (which is all about protecting us from future harm) is to project to the subconscious 'Whoa! Love hurts!' This may then develop into a program to avoid situations associated with 'love' relationships. Then, when you grow up and get into a romantic relationship, you may push that special someone away when they say, 'I love you,' because of that survival program. Once you discover the survival self has the program, and when it began, it can be changed with belief work.

I don't know the circumstances of your birth and early development, but if you were traumatized, there is a good chance that you're going to live your life in worry and stress. You are not going to live the same way as someone that was loved and nurtured. You are going to be in survival mode. But many people are in survival mode and are still motivated by the higher self. They might be terrified to move forward in life, but their higher self pushes them onwards regardless.

Because they are terrified, though, their survival self will try to block them from doing whatever it takes to move forward, even if they know it is their path. So they may end up getting sick right before they do it. But because their higher self is pushing them to do it anyway, there is a battle. I don't know how many people have this type of battle going on, but I suspect it is many. I have also experienced this battle from time to time because part of my life is driven by my higher self, and my forward motion is unstoppable, but my survival self then whines about the situation. So I do my best to motivate myself with different programs. One of these programs I use is, 'I work for the good of the family.' This keeps me working.

If we can shift and change programs, the survival self will feel safe. If the survival self feels safe, we can enact more of the influence of the higher self to create virtues more easily.

For instance, if the virtue of patience is needed, the higher self will bring difficult people who will teach patience. But if every aspect is connected to the higher self then the path to virtues is much easier.

2. THE UNDERCURRENT SELF

The undercurrent is the problem-solver for the brain and at times for the spirit soul. We need the undercurrent part of us to push us forward. It creates situations to fill the need and solves problems. For instance, if a doctor tells someone they have two months to live, it is the undercurrent that says, 'Ah-ha? Want to bet?' If someone says, 'You will never succeed,' it is the undercurrent part of the brain that is activated and says, 'Ah-ha? Want to bet?' And the person goes on to succeed in life.

If someone wants to get even, wreak revenge or punish, this is the undercurrent attempting to solve a problem from the past. The undercurrent doesn't know it is after revenge. To the undercurrent, its actions are simply fixing a problem. One way to find if the undercurrent is influencing a situation is to ask, 'What do I get out of this problem, and what is the motivation for it?'

Depending on the situation, your undercurrent may be working for or against you. You may have a dangerous combination if the negative undercurrent starts running the conscious mind. An example of this is when someone becomes so bent on revenge that the undercurrent starts to plan it out and act on it. But if the conscious mind has enough control and is consciously aware of the subconscious, the person's life is in balance. This means that the undercurrent won't have the opportunity to add unneeded drama.

The undercurrent can be redirected by the balanced conscious mind and by realizing that everything is a manifestation, and the problem can be solved differently.

Healers can help others to get well by showing them what they are doing subconsciously with an option to do something else. As you listen to the client, you can tell them, 'We can shift that.' This makes you a better healer because it teaches discernment.

SELF-BELIEF WORK

The best way to sort out the difference between the different aspects of the belief levels is through self-belief work, which will show you what you are doing subconsciously. If you can identify what your undercurrent is up to, you can learn to know the difference between your higher self and the Creator.

The undercurrent is trying to work for you, even when it might seem to be working against you. It may take many years for the undercurrent to create some scenarios and situations. We may not realize that our actions might be influenced by a problem in the past that the undercurrent considers to be *'unfinished business.'*

For example, I once had a large store with a huge sign saying, 'Vianna's Nature's Path.' I called it that because of a trademark issue over the original name I once used called 'Nature's Path.'

I moved the store closer to the new institute, so the students had better access to the shop and also put in a coffee bar. The new store was smaller than the old one, and I was stuck with the giant sign that I no longer needed. Generally, you can sell an old sign back to the sign-makers so that they can reuse it, but I refused to do this. I was attached to the old sign and didn't want to let it go, so I put it behind the new store. Eventually, my children told me to do some belief work about the old sign. So when I got the chance, I sat down with myself to do some self-belief work about why I was so attached to the sign.

The best way I have found to do self-belief work isn't to ask myself a bunch of questions but to go up and ask the Creator, so I asked:

- 'When did this begin?' (survival self)

- 'What do I get out of it?' (undercurrent self)

- 'What is my attachment to this sign?'

- 'Why am I fighting so hard to keep it?'

When I asked these questions, the Creator showed me the reason instantly, and I found that my attachment to the sign began long ago when I was married to my third husband, and our relationship was difficult.

When I proposed divorce, he levied a threat toward my family and me: 'If you leave me, I will destroy your business, I will destroy your children and then if you are still alive, I will kill you.' Apparently, I believed him and postponed the action for a few months, filling out the divorce papers when I felt braver.

When I found out this was where the attachment began, I thought it was interesting and asked, 'Creator, what did I get out of having the sign?'

Immediately it was clear. Every day, my ex-husband drove past that sign. He couldn't miss it because it was close to him on one of the busiest streets in the town. He loved metaphysical stores and could never come in, but every day it would be impossible for him to ignore. It was a message to him that said, 'I'm still here.' But what I was really saying was, 'I'm still standing.'

I waited 10 years to put up that sign to make sure he knew I wasn't 'destroyed' by him, and I could make it on my own. They say that the best revenge is success, and my undercurrent self worked on this problem for many years and decided to fix it. On some level, I was trying to feel safe because I felt so helpless and afraid at the time. But my undercurrent wasn't afraid; it was simply waiting to take action.

At first, I thought, *Well, that was kind of clever. I am driving him crazy.* Then I couldn't believe that this was my motivation. Did I need to do that anymore? The Creator told me it was a waste of time.

Please understand, I am not angry with my undercurrent. I want you to know that I was delighted on some level to realize my undercurrent went through so much work to put up a huge sign because I realized something very important: I could put that same determination to work for me in my life. Once I learned this about myself, I knew I didn't need to be motivated this way anymore.

I realized my undercurrent was changing problems before and after that. The hidden motivations of other things that I did began to come clear, and it opened up a deeper level of belief work.

To show you how powerful the undercurrent is, I'd like to share something else from my experience. Before I moved from Idaho, I had put up a giant advertisement in the airport at Idaho

Falls that says, 'Founding place of ThetaHealing,' with my picture on it. Since we have moved to Montana, my daughter Bobbi asked me if I wanted to take down the advertisement. But I told her, 'Nope. I want my clients and friends in Idaho to know I'm still standing and to thank them for being there at the beginning of ThetaHealing.'

THE NEGATIVE UNDERCURRENT

A good example of how the undercurrent works negatively is illustrated by the experience of one of my clients, a woman who developed a serious illness. I did belief work with her, and she got better, but the disease came back two years later, and she contacted me again.

During the reading, I could see the disease was getting really bad, so I asked her: 'Okay, if I do a healing on you, what are you going to do if you get completely better? (This is always a great question to ask to see if someone's undercurrent is at work.)

She told me, 'Oh, I don't want to become completely better. My husband cheated on me with my best friend and left me. After that, I got sick, and he came back to take care of me. If it is the last thing that I do, he is going to pay for what he did by taking care of me for the rest of my life.'

What is the undercurrent reason for her holding on to sickness? She wasn't going to be completely better because her undercurrent self was working against her. It brought her husband back to her, but she still wanted to get revenge on him for cheating on her by being stuck taking care of her while she was sick. She tortured him for 15 years.

Breathing room

Sometimes, the undercurrent helps us to get some breathing room in our lives until we are ready to move on. For example, I did a reading with a client who wanted her divorce to be over.

Vianna: 'How long have you been going through a divorce?'

Woman: 'Longer than it should take. I don't know why.'

Vianna: 'When did you decide to get a divorce?'

Woman: 'It started when he was cruel and mean, and I knew I had to get away.'

This response came from the survival self.

Vianna: 'What do you get out of not letting your divorce be finished?'

Woman: 'If it takes a long time, I don't have to date.'

She was obviously afraid of dating.

Vianna: 'Why are you afraid of dating?'

Woman: 'All my friends think I need a husband. I don't want to date, I'm just not ready. I need to know who I am first. The longer it takes, the more time I have for me.

In this case, the client's undercurrent was subconsciously pushing her to take a long time with her divorce so that she could not date.

Control

In another session, the undercurrent was attempting to fix my client's problems with his needy siblings, but it meant submitting to his controlling mother, which was making him unhappy.

Vianna: 'What would you like to work on?'

Man: 'My mother is living with me, and she is driving me crazy.'

Vianna: 'What are you getting out of your mother living with you?'

Man: 'I am not getting anything out of it. She is driving me crazy.'

Vianna: 'Just think about it for a minute. What good are you getting out of her living with you?

He thought about it for a while before speaking.

Man: 'My mother was the most controlling person I ever knew. She controlled me my whole life, and now she is older, she lives with me, and I control her life. My brothers and sister avoid coming to see me and borrowing money because they hate her.

This told me that his undercurrent was both helping and hindering him, so I gave him the following downloads:

- 'Would you like to understand your mother?'

- 'Would you like to know that this part of your life is completed?'

- 'Would you like to know that you can say no to your brothers and sisters?'

These downloads were designed to clear the past and to help him understand his mother; otherwise, the situation wouldn't change positively and healthily for both of them.

Now his conscious mind was able to recognize the need for change, and it all started with one question: 'What did you get out of it?'

Abuse

When I was a young mother, I was watching *The Oprah Winfrey Show* as she interviewed a woman who had been abused as a child. As I listened to this woman tell her story, I thought, *'That is nothing. If that is abuse, then what happened to me was much worse.'*

That was when I realized what had happened to me was abuse and wasn't 'normal.' When I was younger, it was normal to me, but you had better believe that my undercurrent knew it wasn't. By the time I was 29, I was in a course that trained me to be a nuclear security guard, determined that I was never going to be hurt again. After that, I could defend myself. This decision as a mother of three had to come from my undercurrent.

Why did I do that?

I was on a mat fighting with men nearly twice my size, shooting pistols and M16s. In the end, I took another path entirely, but I still finished the course so that I would never have to be a victim again. Our undercurrent pushes us forward to solve what it considers problems even if it takes 30 years or more.

THE GENETIC UNDERCURRENT

The following belief work session is a good example of how genetic programs influence different aspects.

Vianna: 'What would you like to work on?'

Woman: 'I hate my husband.'

Vianna: 'Why do you hate your husband?'

Woman: 'He is angry with me because I work all the time.'

Vianna: 'Do you work all the time?'

Woman: 'Yes, but it's my career. I must work.'

Vianna: 'All the time?'

Woman: 'Yes, if I want to succeed.'

Vianna: 'So there is no time for your husband.'

Woman: 'Our biggest problem is that my work is the most important thing.'

Vianna: 'When did this begin?'

Woman: 'I don't know, it's always been there.'

Vianna: 'Close your eyes and go up to the Seventh Plane and ask the Creator when it began.'

Woman: 'I asked, and it's been there for hundreds of years. You must succeed, you must work, you must be successful as a family, it has always been this way.'

Vianna: 'Okay. Ask the Creator how does this motivate you? What did your family get from this?'

Woman: 'They were guaranteed survival, and they didn't have to spend time together as a couple. This meant they would always stay married.'

Vianna: 'Can you have time for your husband and still work and succeed?'

Woman: 'No, because he would really know me. Love is not real – only the need to survive.'

Vianna: 'Would you like to shift this?'

Woman: 'I guess.'

Vianna: 'Let's change this to "This program is complete. I can have success, and I can work and still have love." Do I have your permission to download "What love *feels like* and that you can *have love*"? Then you can let your husband love you, know you, and still be successful.'

Woman: 'Yes.'

Vianna: 'Are you successful?'

Woman: 'Yes, I am very successful. I easily support my family.'

Vianna: 'Did your parents love one another?'

Woman: 'No, but they respected one another. My mother is a doctor, and my father is an engineer.'

Vianna: 'Let's check if you can have love and success.'

She **energy tests** 'no.'

Woman: 'It's wrong for me to have this because my parents will be jealous and angry. They will think that I am dreaming away from my career.'

Vianna: 'Let's show you that this is possible.'

Woman: 'Okay. But where do I start?'

40

Vianna: 'Let's ask the Creator. Okay, this is what I was told. Do I have permission to download you with, "It's safe to have success and still be in love and that the old program has changed, and you can have both love and success"?'

Woman: 'Yes.'

Her aspects were influencing the situation as follows:

- **Her survival self** was influenced by the genetic program of 'I must succeed to survive.'

- **Her undercurrent self** was influenced by the genetic program of 'my marriage stays together if I stay busy.'

- **Her ego self** was influenced by the program of 'life is measured by money.'

- **Her higher self** was longing for love and self-acceptance, and she was longing for the next step.

- **The Creator says:** 'You can have both love and success to become your best.'

Epigenetics

The following belief-work session is an example how psychological stress can make changes in the physical DNA that are passed down to the next generation; this creates a belief system on the genetic level that influences the aspects.

A woman came to my class, and I noticed that she was aggressive with the other students. But intuitively, I knew that underneath it all, she was a kind person, so when I had the chance, I sat down with her to explore this issue.

Vianna: 'What makes you think that you always have to overcorrect and fight all the time?'

Woman: 'I don't know. I watch myself do it, but I don't understand why.'

Vianna: 'But if you did understand it, when did it start?'

Woman: 'For as long as I can remember, it's always been there.'

Vianna: 'Okay, let's talk about your parents.'

Woman: 'My parents have always been very submissive.'

Vianna: 'Okay, do you have any idea why they are that way?'

Woman: 'Well, my grandmother was a Holocaust survivor.'

Vianna: 'How does that affect you?'

Woman: 'I always heard stories about how the families were led to their deaths.'

Vianna: 'Okay, how does the feeling from those stories serve you? What do you get out of it? Touch your arm and close your eyes. Ask the Creator: "What am I getting out of it? What would my ancestors get out of having this belief?"'

She looked at me with her eyes full of tears.

Woman: 'Because they led to their death by only a few soldiers. Nobody fought back, they just could not believe it was happening to them. My grandmother lost many family members that day, and nobody fought back, so I am going to fight. I will never let that happen to my people again.'

Vianna: 'Would you like to know that you can stand up for yourself and that you know when and how? That you know how to say "no" and that you are safe? And you know when it is the right time to say no, the right time to be strong according to the Creator? And that you don't overcorrect so much anymore?'

Woman: 'Yes, I would!'

So the Creator taught her to know what it was like to be safe, but I suggested that she use the Heart-Song Exercise, which I share in the *Advanced ThetaHealing* book, to clear some of the sorrow from her ancestors.

How was her survival self-influencing the situation? With the programs of: 'I have to fight.'

How was her undercurrent influencing the situation? The undercurrent was working on the problem with the programs of: 'I have to correct what happened to my family' and 'It will never happen to us again.'

Her overcorrection was based on a genetic belief system, and her higher self was motivated to make sure that she got the chance to complete her life mission.

A HISTORY BELIEF SYSTEM

If you are working with a client and they begin to talk about another time and place, they may have a history belief that is associated with the situation. The client may say things like, 'I'm afraid people will kill me like they did before.' This is a survival self-energy reaching the survival part of the history level. However, the history level is also connected to the group consciousness. So the belief that 'diseases are incurable' can be a group conscious belief. Here is an example of this:

Vianna: 'What would you like to work on?'

Client: 'I am diabetic, but I never use my insulin or change my diet or lifestyle, and I don't know what is wrong with me.'

Vianna: 'Well, what do you get out of not taking your diabetes medicine?'

Client: 'If I don't take it, I think that I will get better because diabetes is incurable, and I can never get better.'

Vianna: 'What else do you get out of not taking medicine?'

Client: 'I'm trying to make my body heal itself.'

Vianna: 'Okay, how does that serve you?'

Client: 'As long as I have diabetes, I have to take care of myself, so I have a fight going on inside me.'

Vianna: 'What are you going to do about that fight?'

Client: 'I suspect I'm going to have to take care of myself one way or the other.'

How are the aspects influencing the situation?

The survival self is saying: 'Diabetes is incurable,' and 'I don't want it.'

The undercurrent is saying: 'I'm going to have to take care of myself.' The reward to the undercurrent is that as long as the client has diabetes, they are going to have to take care of themselves.

In this situation, the client should be given downloads to teach them how to take care of themselves, such as 'I know how to live without feeling completely helpless.'

For more explanations of belief work, refer to *Digging for Beliefs*.

The ego self

We need the ego part of ourselves to maintain our identity. We should not tell our ego to go away because it's our self-image, but we can keep it from thinking it's better than anyone else. Just as with the undercurrent, the ego is neither good nor bad. Once you understand your undercurrent, it will be much easier to recognize the influences of your ego-self that can be both positive and negative.

I call a negative ego *egotism*. When egotism is expressing itself from the subconscious, it always offers fame and money at the expense of someone else. Someone that is in egotism will say and think things like, 'You must love me' as opposed to 'Do you love me?'

The ego must be redirected toward developing virtues. Virtues give the ego high self-esteem. Virtues help retain your ego as a friend rather than turn it into egotism. When the ego is directed toward positive actions, you are in control. It becomes egotism when you are *controlled by the ego*.

For example, when you start doing readings, you might be unsure and nervous at first wondering if you 'got it right.' In the first reading, the practitioner says things to the client, such as: 'I see something wrong with your shoulder.' The client confirms the reader is right, and this begins to work on the mind of the reader. Because of the truth of this statement, the practitioner does more readings and continues to 'get it right' time after time. Flushed with success, the reader makes the mistake of falling into the trap of egotism. They forget all about the Creator and begin to make statements such as: 'I think you should do this with your life.' The reader may begin to think that it is 'all about them' and forget that the reading is a co-creative process. As long as you remember to simply relay the message from the Creator, all is good.

Many years ago, a woman came into my shop and introduced herself as having a message from the **Council of Twelve**. I said, 'Okay, what is the message?'

She said, 'The Council of Twelve say you have done a great job, but now it is time for me to take over from you.'

Would the Council of Twelve tell her it was her job to take over? Unlikely. There is a Council of Twelve for every soul family, so which one was she talking about? Obviously, she wanted my clients, my shop, and my business. Without hesitation, I told her, 'I'm sorry, but the Creator didn't tell me anything like that.'

This is a good example of someone whose ego self was in egotism. She wasn't channeling anything, although I am sure that she believed what she said, and her egotism thought was that she could convince me.

In my advanced class, I share an exercise to experience the higher self in another person. One student is the client, and the other is the practitioner. The client gives the practitioner a series of questions directed to their higher self. Using the Road Map Meditation to the Creator (*see Introduction, page xiv*), the practitioner connects to the higher self and acts as a go-between for questions and answers.

As two of my students were doing this exercise, a woman in the role of the client asked her higher self why she couldn't find her soul mate and what she needed to do to find them faster. Supposedly talking to the client's higher self, the practitioner replied, 'Your higher self says you have to dye your hair blonde!'

This answer upset the lady who was the client, and she came up to me crying and asked me, 'Does my higher self really want me to dye my hair blonde?'

I told her, 'Of course not. Don't worry about it.'

Do you really think that this woman's higher self-aspect would tell her that? Is her soul mate going to come into her life sooner because she became blonde? I don't think so. Still, I asked her higher self just to make sure, and it hadn't said anything about her hair.

Can you guess what color hair the practitioner had? That's right, blonde! The practitioner was speaking from her egotism and her own experience. She may have genuinely been trying to help the other woman with dark hair, but was obviously being influenced by her ego self. The question that should have been asked of the woman's higher self was, 'Is she ready for her soul mate?' Regardless, it was still the responsibility of the woman getting the reading to go up and find out if the reader was right.

The Higher Self

The higher self keeps everything in perspective. As long as you are embracing your higher aspect, you will get better responses from the universe. Most of the time, we are acting through one or more of the aspects of survival, undercurrent, or ego instead of the higher self.

Your subconscious aspects are connected to your higher self and your higher self connects to your soul, but the higher self still has to go up to the Creator for the highest truth and balance all the aspects. We need our higher self for the growth of our soul.

The goal is to let your higher self run more of your life. The more you allow your higher aspect into your space, the more virtues you will have, and the more you can go through your higher self to the Creator. Unlike the aspects of the first three levels, it *knows* it is part of the Creator.

The belief systems of the higher self are:

- 'I can grow.'

- 'I can learn.'

- 'We are part of the Creator.'

- 'The Creator is part of us.'

Some messages from the Creator would be:

- 'We are all part of the Creator.'

- 'We are all atoms. '

- 'We are all part of the life-force.'

- 'We are all loved.'

- 'We are allowed to connect to this energy.'

The higher self says, '*I* can learn' but the Creator will pull you out of me, me, me, and says '*We* can *all* learn.'

The soul

We are living in the body's life support system which works three-dimensionally. The higher self works from a Third Plane consciousness, connecting to the higher aspect of the soul. But the soul works multidimensionally and isn't completely confined to the body while it is a configuration of all the different levels and aspects. Destiny is the embodiment of the soul's desire to grow. The soul believes that once something is changed, the effect is immediate.

Working with the Aspects

ASPECTS OF DIGGING WORK

It is important to understand that when we do belief work, we are working on all aspects of the levels. However, it is important to recognize which aspects are at work in the levels and how much they influence your life from a subconscious level.

The awareness that your inner aspects may be *influencing* a belief work session doesn't change how you *use* belief work. The practitioner is still working on four levels of belief – core, history, genetic, and soul levels. Still requesting and commanding that beliefs are released and replaced. Still doing digging work the same way – asking the same basic questions in belief work. You are still going up to the Creator before you do belief work to ask for answers and the correct downloads. What we are introducing here is more knowledge of ourselves and how to know the difference between the Creator and other influences. This realization can help you heal.

If for example you go up to the Creator and hear a pure answer like, 'You are part of All That Is,' the survival part of your brain might whisper, 'No I'm not worthy to be part of All That Is.' Obviously, this voice isn't coming from the highest place because you have common sense. Still, you also know that it is time to work on this belief.

Your undercurrent will take this answer from the Creator in a totally different way, as will your ego. If these aspects are in

51

balance, then they will accept the answer in the highest way. If they are unbalanced, then the interpretation will not be.

ASPECT DIGGING

When you use your connection with the Creator in a belief-work session, your time is cut in half because the Creator simply shows you the answer. In this exercise, the reader pretends to be both the practitioner and client with a focus on recognizing the survival self, undercurrent self, ego self, and higher self.

1. To begin the session, think of the problems you are having in your life.

2. Once you have identified what you want to work on, go up to the Seventh Plane using the Road Map Meditation (*see Introduction, page xiv*).

3. Now that you are in the Seventh Plane ask the Creator, 'Where did this begin? Where did this feeling start?' (This question is directed at the Creator to uncover the survival self.) Through the answer, the reader will recognize the survival self and what it is doing.

4. Next, go back to the Seventh Plane using the Road Map Meditation again. Now that you are in the Seventh Plane, ask the Creator, 'What do I get out of this? How is this motivating me? Show me.' Through this answer, the client

recognizes the undercurrent self and what it is doing. (Remember the Creator always has loving energy.)

5.   Next, return to the Seventh Plane using the Road Map Meditation. Now that you are in the Seventh Plane ask the Creator, 'What is my ego creating? What am I achieving from this? Show me.' Through this answer, the reader recognizes the ego self and what it is doing.

Note: If you ask, 'How does this affect me?' this is the ego self speaking.

6.   Next, go to the Seventh Plane using the Road Map Meditation. Now that you are in the Seventh Plane ask the Creator, 'What is my higher self-learning from this? Show me.' Through this answer, the reader recognizes the higher self and what it is doing.

Note: The reader should keep doing the belief work until the motivations of each aspect become apparent, while at all times going to the Creator for the highest answer.

7.   Go to the Seventh Plane using the meditation. Now that you are in the Seventh Plane, ask the Creator, what do you want me to learn? Show me the Creator's perspective.' Through this answer, the client recognizes the Creator. This would be a pure, channeled message. Now the reader should ask the Creator if there is anything else to learn from the experience, what downloads are needed, and what needs to be shifted and changed.

Note: If you ask, 'Creator, what am I doing?' you are connecting to divine energy.

8.   Do you trust the Creator to help you with these issues? Go up and ask the Creator if you trust the Creator.

9.   Ask the Creator, 'Is this is completed?'

After practicing this exercise for the first time, you will begin to recognize the influences of the aspects on your daily life. A **sleep cycle** will give your conscious mind a better idea of what is going on with the subconscious, and it will be easier to recognize what is going on with the four aspects of survival, undercurrent, ego, and higher self.

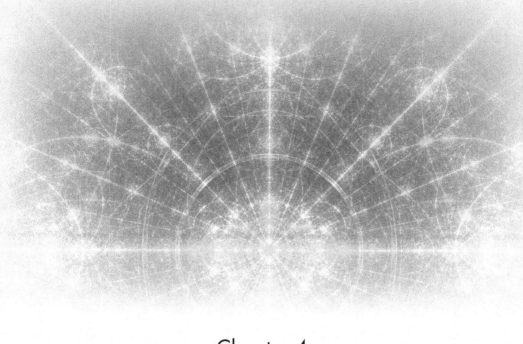

Chapter 4

KNOWING THE DIFFERENCE BETWEEN THE CREATOR AND SELF

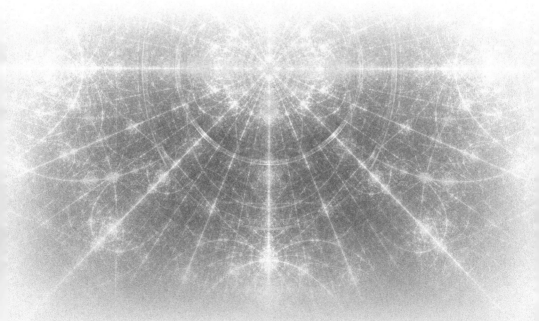

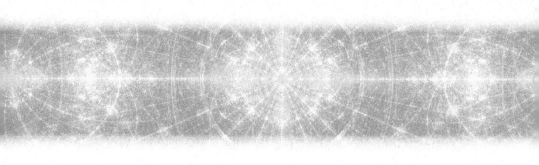

Once you know how to recognize all the aspects in your mind, it is easier to understand your intuition and what messages you are receiving.

Remember, there are always two conversations going on in your head. This is normal, so don't think this is a mental illness of some kind. By the time you talk to the aspects of the survival, undercurrent, and ego selves, you may find you have all kinds of influences in your head.

It is important to ask:

- 'What part of me is this?'

- 'What does it feel like to visit with the Creator? It is the pure energy of intelligence and perfect love.'

It is not uncommon to get many answers when you go up to connect to the Creator.

When you go up to the Creator, ask for the highest truth that your enlightened higher self would get when talking with the Creator. Going up and asking for the highest truth will help you to get better answers. If you are not sure that the answer is right, keep asking for the 'highest truth' until you know it is the most intelligent, loving answer.

Fear is one thing that can block you from the highest truth. The answer from the Creator is always the most intelligent, loving answer and is never laced with fear or egotism.

BEING CONSCIOUS OF THE ANSWERS

If you really want to know what is going on in your head, be conscious of the answers you receive to your questions to the Creator.

A good example of this is with one student who thought I didn't like her because I didn't stop to give her a hug. Offended and hurt, she texted me and said, 'I asked the Creator why you didn't like me and was told, "It doesn't matter anyway, it is your teacher's problem. Anyone that you trust hurts you anyway."'

Obviously, this answer didn't come from the Creator, because I like her very much, So, I wrote back and told her to go up again and ask the same question. When she did, she replied that she received the answer, 'As long as I keep my distance, I will be safe. I can only count on myself.'

This is a classic reply from her undercurrent self. So then I texted her, 'Why do you believe that? What do you get out of having that belief? Is that really what you think?'

She wrote back, 'Yes, this is what I believe.'

So I asked her, 'Why do you feel that way? Once you know why you feel that way, go up to the Creator again.'

She texted back and said, 'I am better than you anyway. I will create my own stuff.'

This was obviously her egotism talking to her, and the whole interaction from start to finish went like this:

First, I gently told her that I did like her, and she was very special. Then I told her to ask the Creator her question:

Question: 'Why doesn't my teacher like me?'

Survival self: 'It doesn't matter, it is the teacher's problem. Anyone I trust hurts me anyway.'

Question: 'Why doesn't my teacher like me?'

Undercurrent self: 'As long as I keep my distance from them, I will be safe. I can only count on myself.'

This is because the survival self believes that anyone this person trusts hurts them.

Question: 'Why doesn't my teacher like me? How does this motivate me?'

Negative ego: 'I am better than them anyway. I will create my own stuff.'

This response by the negative ego is because the survival self believes that anyone they trust hurts them, and the undercurrent is trying to solve the problem.

These answers mean that the student is in their own space and not talking to the Creator. I found this was a fairly common scenario because there is always someone that has experienced having their feelings hurt by a teacher and so are terrified of trusting anyone or anything. Each time I encouraged her to ask again for the highest answer.

Question: 'Why doesn't my teacher like me? What am I learning from this?'

Higher self: 'My teacher loves her students. What are they trying to teach me, Creator?'

At last, she discovered the real answer.

Question: 'Why doesn't my teacher like me?'

The Creator would respond with love and truth.

The Creator: 'Your teacher is tired. What can you do for them? What can you learn from them? Truly they have blessed your life.'

The Creator would pull you out of the space that is about yourself and show you the answer from a place of perfect love. The Creator always answers from this place, which means that many of the messages given to practitioners and teachers of ThetaHealing are influenced by the inner aspects instead of being influenced by the Creator. One of the reasons that we go up and connect to the Creator is so that we don't get caught up in the influences of our brain. If there is any residue of fear in the communication, the answer isn't coming from the Creator.

When you go up and talk to the Creator, use the following guides:

- Keep asking until you receive the highest answer.

- You have to navigate through your mind. The highest answer might not be the first one. It will, however, be the clearest, highest, least selfish, and kindest answer. It will make your heart warm. What would the highest intelligence and love say to you?

- Common sense is important. Let your conscious mind make the decision and ask: 'Is this what the Creator would tell me?'

- The voice is wrong if it is negative. Don't listen to it. Anytime it says things like 'you can't do healing' or 'you're nothing,' it has the wrong energy.

- The subconscious solves problems of the past with the undercurrent. Sometimes it overcorrects and needs the conscious mind to redirect it. You must understand your true motivation as it relates to your undercurrent, or it can keep you trapped.

We need all of the aspects, but they also have to be in balance. When you go up and see what's running your life, your job is to consciously balance things in the subconscious.

DOWNLOADS

The following downloads can help you understand your subconscious self better.

'I know how to understand myself.'

'I am ready to understand my subconscious mind.'

'I know how to let my conscious mind run my subconscious.'

'I know how to understand my survival self.'

'I know how to understand my undercurrent self.'

'I know how to understand my ego self.'

'I know how to understand my higher self.'

'I know what it feels like for my aspects to work together.'

'I know how to allow the Creator to teach through me.'

'I know what it feels like to have wisdom flow to me.'

'I know how to give love and attention to others because they are coming from the Creator.'

'I know how to trust the Creator.'

•••

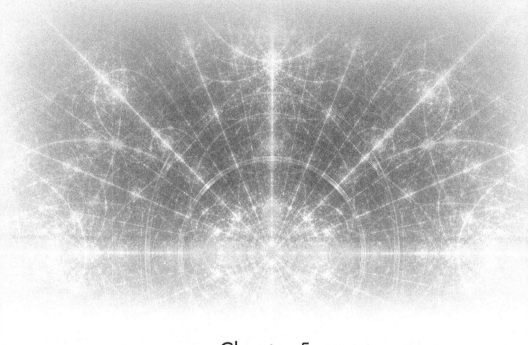

Chapter 5

UNDERSTANDING MESSAGES FROM THE CREATOR

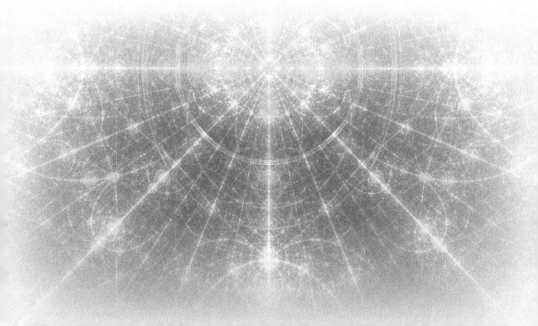

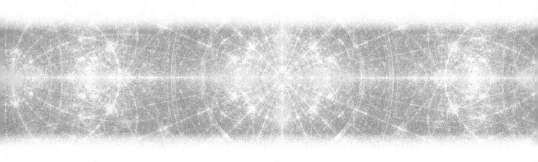

If you are in harmony with creation, you will receive messages from the universe, but only if you pay attention. As a psychic, you will get messages in many ways. It might be through the words of a song that you receive inspiration when you need it the most. Some people receive messages in their dreams, generally in the early hours of the morning (1–3 a.m.). It is not uncommon to wake up and think, 'I can't remember everything about the dream, but I know the message was really important. What happened?'

Not to worry, you will keep getting the dream until you remember it. This is normal. If you go to sleep and you feel that people are working on you, this is also normal. All you have to do as it relates to night work is to know that you are okay. However, if you are awake and you think your TV is talking to you, telling you to scrub your kitchen floor, then you might have to worry and question your sanity.

We all receive divine inspiration if we are open to hearing it. One of the messages some people get is that we are all part of the Creator. While this message is a good one, it still depends on how it is interpreted. If someone is in survival mode, it may be that this will trigger survival beliefs on a genetic level. Some of these beliefs might be 'it is wrong to think we are all part of the Creator' or 'I could be killed' from the history level. The undercurrent belief might be, 'I am not good enough to be part of the Creator.' The egotism would say 'the Creator is me; I am the Creator, I am the most important, worship me. I am better than anyone. I will prove I am better than anyone else. I will show them!' But really the message should be 'we are all part of the energy that moves in all things. You are part of the whole.'

Example Message: 'You are part of the Creator.'

Survival: 'It is wrong to think I am part of the Creator. I could be killed.'

Undercurrent: 'I am not good enough to be part of the super-conscious of the Creator. I must be feared, or I must hide so no one will really see me.'

Egotism: 'The Creator is me; I am the Creator, I am the most important, worship me. I can be better than anyone. I will prove I am better. I'll show them, I will create something. I'm as good as them.'

Higher self: The soul says, 'I can make a difference. I can learn, I can grow and help everyone I can. We are all part of God.

The Creator would respond with love and truth, such as, 'We are all connected to the energy of All That Is. We are all atoms; we are all part of the life-force. We are all loved and allowed to connect to this energy.' The Creator would pull you out of a space that is about yourself and show you the answer with love.

You may get a message that you will work with a famous movie star, but your ego says, 'No, that is just too conceited – to think that I would work with someone that important.' Obviously, your ego lacks confidence, and you disregarded the message because you didn't think you were worthy enough. You may have stopped an opportunity to help someone that needs it. After all, movie stars have some very weird, cool entertaining challenges to work through just like everyone else.

As this relates to the ego self, there is a difference between being confident and being self-centered. But there is a difference between being centered in yourself and only thinking about yourself. We are supposed to love ourselves without being self-centered, love others, love a significant other, and love the Creator. To be balanced, you should love yourself 40 percent and everyone else 60 percent. This love thing is tricky but necessary to get clear answers.

Which self are you connecting to when you get a message in your mind? For instance, if you were taking a trip to teach ThetaHealing and the message that comes is 'something is wrong with the airplane,' this is likely your survival self because this message is about fear.

Your undercurrent would get you out of going on a trip differently. Your undercurrent would begin questioning why you were going on the trip in the first place and try to figure a way so that you don't have to go.

Since your undercurrent knows that the way you have avoided going to places was to get sick, you may find you get sick right before you get on the airplane. Your negative ego would tell you things such as, 'I am going to be magnificent; I am going to be worshipped in the class I am going to teach.' The higher self would say, 'You will be safe on the trip, and this is part of your divine timing.' If the message came from the Creator, the message wouldn't have any fear or ego. The message would be something like 'Relax. It's going to all be okay.'

Your higher self is very knowledgeable because it is connected to your soul. Your soul is part of God, the Creator, but there is nothing like going directly to the universal spirit that animates and binds all things in existence.

I once had a client with a problem. She couldn't figure out why she always burned the food when she was cooking. For five years, she didn't know why she was burning her husband's dinner until she went up and connected to the Creator and asked, 'When did this start? Why am I burning his dinner? Am I still angry with him?'

The Creator told her, 'It started when he hurt your feelings. He is going to eat burned dinners until you forgive him. You are still angry with him. Once your anger is completed, you can move on.'

Part of her brain was still trying to solve the problem by burning his dinner. She thought to herself, 'It would be nice to not eat burned dinner. Maybe I should forgive him.'

It never occurred to this woman that she was burning her husband's dinner because her subconscious had not reached forgiveness.

•••

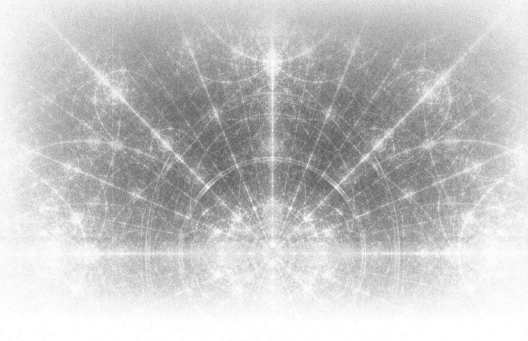

Chapter 6

INTUITIVE MESSAGES FROM THE CREATOR

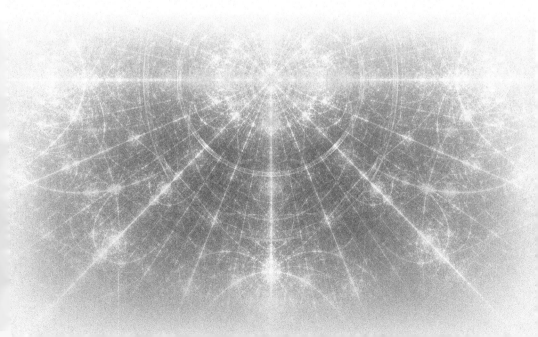

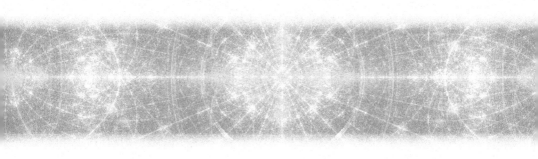

It takes good judgment to receive pure information from the Creator. This is the judgment of how to listen and use the information once you have the message. This requires faith in the message from the Creator. Once you know how to use the information, it is important to take action, as the following stories from my past illustrate.

CHARLIE'S RESTAURANT

When I first started my business, I had an experience that taught me to listen when I got a message from the Creator. One night I was working in my little shop, and I was ready to go home. I turned off all the lights and then I heard the Creator say, 'You can't leave. Sit down and be still.'

I replied, 'Oh no, I'm okay.'

But the Creator said, 'Sit down. There is danger outside.'

So I sat down and waited for an hour.

Then I heard, 'Everything is okay. Go home.'

The messages had such a powerful energy that there was no doubt in my mind that I had to listen.

The next day I was in my office doing a massage, and suddenly, the fire department came beating on my door. I opened the door, and the fireman said, 'We have to evacuate the building now! There is a bomb!'

At the time, I thought this was ridiculous because nobody makes bombs in Idaho, especially the conservative town of Idaho Falls. Nevertheless, I got my client off the table, and we went outside to find out what was going on.

In this building, there was a restaurant, a beauty parlor, a metaphysical store, and my office in the back of the store. The restaurant was called Charlie's Restaurant. That day, the people who ran the beauty shop smelled gasoline and called the fire department, which found that a bomb had been constructed on the rooftop. They defused the bomb and called the police who investigated and arrested Charlie, who eventually went to prison.

Apparently, Charlie was losing money and wanted the insurance money in the event of a fire. So the night before, thinking everyone had gone home, Charlie winched large barrels of gasoline to the top of the building, and connected a makeshift igniter and timer to blow up the next night when everyone went home. If I had walked out that night, I would have run right into his bombmaking fiasco. What was important was that I listened to the voice and this was a good lesson for me.

INTUITIVE ANATOMY IN NEW ZEALAND

I once did an intuitive anatomy class in Rotorua, New Zealand, for some indigenous Māori folks and other New Zealanders. We stayed in a hotel room on the first floor with sliding doors to the outside.

One night I was told to move to a different room in the hotel. The message was clear: 'Move, or you are going to get robbed.'

I told Guy that we had to move to another room. Irritated, he said he didn't want to move. That day a water pipe broke in our room, and the hotel moved us one level up to another room.

Guy laughed and said, 'You got your way after all!'

The next night everyone on the first floor got robbed when they were out to dinner, and our host was one of these people, which made me very sad.

HURRICANE SANDY

When I was doing a seminar in upstate New York, I heard about a hurricane called Sandy that had developed in the

Atlantic and was swirling toward the coast. I had just finished the seminar and drove back to New York City to fly home. I wanted to extend my flight for a couple of days and show my daughter Brandy New York City. Then I was told by the Creator to fly out to avoid the storm, and by this time, I had learned to listen.

In this seminar, many of my coordinators had come from other countries. I told them all to fly out early, and to their credit, they listened to me. But my friend that lives in NYC argued with me saying, 'These storms threaten New York regularly but they have never hit and this one won't either.' He told everyone that I was coming from fear and not to listen to me, but my other coordinators knew better.

We all got early flights and made it out before the storm hit. One hour after the last coordinator flew out, the airport shut down because of the storm, and no one left the city.

For the first time in recent memory Manhattan was hit by a hurricane that caused a great deal of damage. Had I stayed, I would have been delayed for days. Hurricane Sandy forced the cancellation of 9,250 flights grounding 810,000 passengers, causing over $50 billion in damage in 24 states. The hardest-hit areas were along the New Jersey coastline and into Long Island. In NYC, the storm closed subway stations, caused fires, and closed the New York Stock Exchange. Sandy shut down multiple airports and train stations across the Northeast. The rain, snow, and winds from Sandy left over eight million people without power from the Atlantic coast to the Great Lakes, and some homes in New York and New Jersey were without power for weeks after the storm. Hurricane Sandy claimed the lives of 147 people.

The moral of these stories? You have to be able to listen to the Creator and take the appropriate action.

ENHANCING COMMUNICATION WITH THE CREATOR

The following practices help open the crown chakra and increase communication with the Creator:

- You should have energy coming into your crown chakra all the time, so there is constant communication with the Creator.

- Gather energy into your body and gently push it up toward the crown. If necessary, start the process over again. This has little to do with rolling your eyes or straining. This is not the kind of push as when you go to the bathroom. Just imagine a gentle upward push.

- Violet Light therapy may help to open the crown chakra and create a connection. If you lie under violet light, it will improve your focus for phone readings.

- Infrared light therapy helps to detoxify the body and focus the mind. It helps to get oxygen to the cells and balance your hormones.

- If the answer from the Creator has a negative or fearful response, cancel it and go higher. The energy of the Creator is the perfect and pure energy of love and intelligence. If you are going up and get an answer that doesn't feel as though it is from this place of purity, then you need to imagine yourself going higher and ask: 'What is the highest answer?' As you start to do this, you will realize that you are going up through the levels of the planes of existence to the Seventh Plane.

- If you want clear messages from the Creator, you must ask yourself some questions to know yourself. The next step is to do self-work with the Creator. The best way to do self-work is to go up to the Creator and ask, 'When did the issue start? What am I getting out of it? What am I learning from it?'

- If the message isn't the most loving evolved energy, then it probably isn't the Creator.

- The clarity of the messages you receive depends on how much you practice going up and connecting to the Creator.

ASPECT BELIEF WORK WITH ANOTHER PERSON

It is important to develop the ability to do belief work with the Creator. But it is also useful to help someone else do belief work with the Creator. This exercise is to get someone used to working with the Creator and requires two people: One person is the client and the other the practitioner. It's important to note the following:

1. The practitioner teaches the client to connect to the Creator to work with the aspects.

2. The practitioner has the client ask the Creator belief-work questions for themselves.

3. The practitioner then tells the client to go up to the Seventh Plane each time they ask the Creator a question.

4. Throughout the exercise, the practitioner psychically witnesses what the client is doing.

Here is an example of dialogue of doing aspect belief work with another person:

Practitioner: 'What issue are you experiencing at the moment?'

Client: *'I always sabotage my relationships with people I love.'*

Now that the practitioner has identified what the client wants to work on, the practitioner tells the client to go to the Seventh Plane to ask the Creator this question:

Practitioner: 'I want you to go up to the Creator and find out when this began.'

The client takes themselves to the Seventh Plane and asks the Creator and gets an answer. 'It began when I was a child.'

When the client has the answer, the practitioner asks the client, 'What would you do next? What is the next step?'

Practitioner: 'Go up and ask the Creator what you are getting out of it. How does it serve you?'

Client: *The Creator told me If I sabotage my relationships, I will never be hurt by someone I love.'*

Practitioner: 'Ask the Creator what you are learning from this.'

Client: *'The Creator tells me that I am learning that I can love others, and they can love me.'*

The practitioner tells the client to ask the Creator to give them the necessary downloads or change the beliefs that are needed.

As you have noticed, it is important to train yourself to listen. Going directly to the Creator can cut digging time by half.

●●●

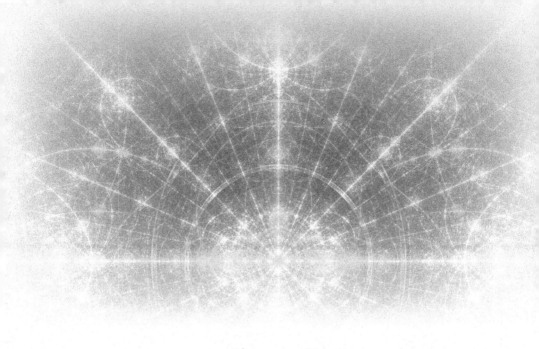

Chapter 7

SORTING
THINGS OUT

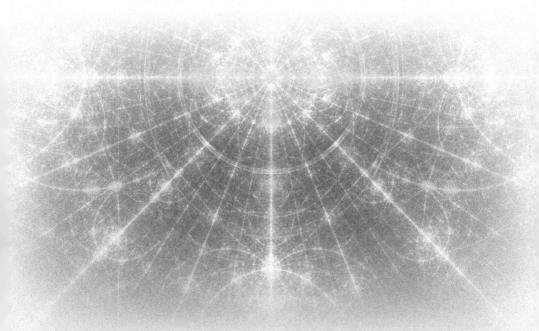

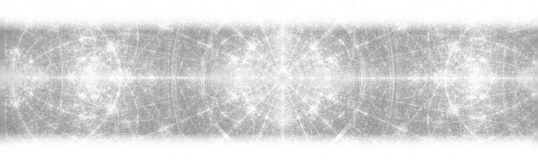

In this chapter, we will explore what things can BLOCK us from receiving clear messages from the Creator.

EGOTISM

We have discussed the pitfalls of egotism already, but here I'd like to explore the topic in more depth and why it is so important for the reader to keep their ego out of a session.

I learned this in the early years when I let a few people do readings in my shop. I could see that that they had psychic abilities, but for some reason, they couldn't leave their egotism out of it. The problem was they were projecting their own issues on the clients.

One psychic told all their clients that they were gay, but they just didn't know it yet. So who was gay? The reader was gay!

I had another psychic doing readings that told everyone they were headed for a relationship breakup. This person actually believed what they were saying but who was headed for a breakup? The reader!

If you tell five or six people a day that they are gay or that their spouses are going to leave them, there is a problem. I had to let the readers go because they couldn't tell the difference between the truth of their ego and divine truth.

RULE OR LEAD

One of the things that keeps us from moving forward to get clear answers from the Creator is the ego wanting to rule others instead of wanting to lead. Ruling and leading are two different things.

The ego of a ruler screams: 'I know what is best for them. I want to rule!' The ruler wants to be worshiped, and the leader wants to lead with inspiration and love to make a better world. A leader pulls everyone working together, and a ruler wants everyone to do exactly what they say.

The difference between ruling and leading is easy to see in the world's politicians. Some government officials get obsessed with the need to be worshiped and rule with an iron fist – the 'might makes right' mentality.

Wanting to rule others stops anyone from getting clear answers from the Creator because it is against the Law of Free Agency.

What is true in politics is also true in teaching or doing readings. The reader or teacher must lead others, not attempt to rule or control them. You can't make someone love or worship you. Love happens naturally. If you want to work with other people, with the world, and work with the Creator, then you need to connect with God. But If you want people to worship you, this is the wrong modality. Being a ruler and trying to control everyone will stop you from getting clear messages.

POWER

As you heal others, you're going to get energy from the Creator, which is actually powerful. So if you're afraid of your own power, you have to remember it's actually the *life-force of the Creator* that is the power. Any power must be used wisely. The fear of power can stop clear answers as can the obsession for power.

PRIMAL INSTINCT

Instinct is considered to be behavior-based genetic factors that are acted on without the influence of life learning or experience. As humans, we have developed primal instincts, and a good example of this is when one person is sexually attracted to another. All of his or her instincts go off, telling them that the other person would be a good mate, and for this reason, they are likely to agree to date even if they don't know the other person, because of the optimism of his or her instincts. But when they are on the date, they have a conversation and may realize that the other person isn't what he or she expected.

This is one way that pheromones can create an attraction purely from primal instinct. The body thinks someone is physically acceptable, but the mind must be attracted as well. Primal instincts must be tempered with wisdom.

ISSUES OF THE FOUR RS

Four emotional reactions that block us from receiving clear messages are resentment, regret, rejection, and revenge. They all take up a lot of mental space and, in some instances, work within the undercurrent. Regret can stop you from moving forward, and rejection is not always taken well by the undercurrent. Your undercurrent can get stuck on these programs and can have a difficult time moving past them.

The more of these negative programs are cleared, the more the undercurrent can be redirected to work on someone's behalf. Remember, the undercurrent is not the enemy, only a part of who we are. You can have a lot of fun, just understanding yourself. Once something is learned from regrets or resentment, then the wisdom goes to the higher self that is connected to the soul.

The inherent danger of falling into the four Rs – resentment, regret, rejection, and revenge – is illustrated by the following anecdote, Tommy the Leprechaun.

Many years ago, I started my office doing readings, massage, and naturopath consultations in Idaho Falls, Idaho. I wanted my office to be a place where people could come to sit and rest, so I left tea out for anyone that wanted it when I was doing a session. It didn't take long for all the people in the neighborhood to come in, sit down, and help themselves to tea. So, when I walked out of my session, there was always someone drinking tea. Needless to say, I went through a lot of tea.

Some of these people who came in for tea were homeless window washers. They'd do a good job washing my windows and do a mediocre job on the neighbors. They'd tell me, 'You don't have anything. You're like us. We'll clean your windows because you're nice.' Tommy, the Leprechaun, was one of these traveling vagrants and came every year to Idaho Falls for the warm months.

Then one day, one of my clients told me that Tommy was in town, and I asked them to introduce me. Tommy was one of those magical characters that you only meet once in a lifetime, and he looked just like a Leprechaun.

He was just a little fella that always wore green and had these big, expressive eyes much like a deer. He handed out a card that said, 'one free wish: Tommy the Leprechaun' and tied balloons. He would sing and play his guitar, and people would give him money. (He really did look like a leprechaun.)

As I got to know him, he told me stories about how he had been a tunnel rat in the Vietnam War because he was so small. He had only four fingers because of a bomb in one of the tunnel excursions. The war had made him so resentful of the government that he became a street person. He would make enough every day for his dinner every night. He would get a new set of clothes at the Salvation Army every three days, always green. He would come into my office with a guitar to sing songs, and we became fast friends. I came to love Tommy.

One night we were talking, and it began to rain, so I let him stay in my office. When I got to work the next morning, he had stolen my window cleaner. When I saw him later that day, I said, 'Tommy, you stole my window cleaner!' He smiled at me and said, 'I knew you wouldn't mind.'

We'd visit, but he never asked me for money (probably because he knew I didn't have any at the time). I came to know he had emphysema, so I'd give him herbal teas for it. Our friendship lasted for two summers because he would leave before winter came along.

Then I met Blake, who was to become my third husband. Appearances were very important to him, and when I walked into a store with him and saw Tommy, I went to talk to Tommy, and he stopped me saying, 'You can't talk to that person in public! He is a vagrant!' He grabbed my arm and pulled me away. But Tommy saw me walk away, and I will never forget the pain in his eyes because he had been rejected by me.

A few days went by, and I saw Tommy on the street, and I stopped to talk to him. He told me he was leaving town and I gave him a ride to the bus stop. The feeling between us was different, and I knew I had ruined our friendship. I had walked away from a friend. I apologized, and he said he understood, but this just made me feel worse.

His feelings were too badly hurt, and no matter what abuse had ever happened to me, the pain of that moment was so bad that it was one of the worst things in my life. I had gone out of my way to walk away and hurt this innocent, perfect soul. I never saw Tommy again.

I held on to that regret for years, and I promised myself I would never let it happen again. I've never forgotten that absolute pain of regret. I have done my best to never make someone feel less than another. One night a few years later, I had a dream that Tommy was looking in my refrigerator for something to eat.

What I learned from Tommy was that everyone matters. Everyone is important, no matter what anyone thinks. I had to forgive myself for Tommy, but only when I was sure that it wouldn't happen again.

What is that one thing that you may have done to hurt someone's feelings a long time ago? What things have you done in your life you regret? If you have made a difficult decision and still regret it, the undercurrent goes in circles over it. For instance, your undercurrent will go in circles if you missed your chance to be in love, and you might believe that you will never have the chance again. Thank goodness I am married to Guy!

Releasing regrets

When you reach 50 years old, your brain does something really amazing – it works! Then when you look back at your life, half of your regrets are gone because you realize, 'Oh, I was a child when I did that' or 'Oh, I was only 30 when that happened.' The next step is to come to the realization that throughout your life, you may be listening to the higher self more than you realize. You may have made more right decisions than wrong ones.

Everyone should be proud of what they have accomplished and forgive themselves for what they have not. Clearing revenge, resentment, rejection, and regret help us to know the difference between the planes of existence and our connection to the Creator. If you could see your past decisions from the Creator's perspective, you might not have as much regret as you think.

Of all the creatures in the universe (that we know of), it is only humans that look back and relive the past. If you regret something, find out what you can learn from it. If you can learn something from it, you will stop replaying the regret over and over again. Replaying past regrets keeps you from moving forward. As you find what you learned from it, you will start to like yourself. For every time you regret something, your undercurrent will try to fix it as you say to yourself, 'I will never do that again,' so that you never do it again!

If you want to keep people away from you, resentment works well, while rejection can cause you to go in circles as well. If you were harshly rejected as a child, your undercurrent is going to attempt to correct it as an adult. For instance, if your mother rejected you, you might spend your whole life chasing her for that love. Another correction from the undercurrent might be to completely reject her.

Regret and depression

All the aspects of the levels must work together in balance and harmony. For instance, the survival self is aware of specific foods that the body needs for survival. It sends messages to the body in the way of cravings for foods that have the needed vitamins, amino acids, or minerals.

If the survival self is well balanced, it will make sure the body has everything it needs. But there can be disharmony if the other aspects are not sending the right messages to one another. If the undercurrent is going in circles, it can affect the functions of the survival self.

A good example of this is when the undercurrent self is going in circles, unable to let go of regret. One of the things that can cause depression is when the undercurrent constantly lives with regret and can't figure out the answer to a problem. When this happens, the mind constantly goes in circles and doesn't rest, which can cause the survival self to go into emergency mode. This constant emergency mode can block the survival self from releasing serotonin, and other vital chemicals that the brain and body need in order to maintain balance, and depression is the result. This is why the undercurrent needs to find what has been learned from the regret and let it go.

Our mind has to practice virtues to be balanced. If someone has a balanced ego, they have a positive self-image and generally don't develop depression because they don't live in regret. Without regret, we can establish a balanced ego, and the aspects stay balanced too. Remember, a balanced ego and high self-esteem help the body function as it should. If you release issues of regret with belief work, you are going to get what I call a 'good ego.'

The more someone consciously knows what they want to achieve, the more they have a connection with the higher self. The better connection with the higher self, the more balance there is in all the different belief levels, and the stronger and healthier they become. All the aspects have to be balanced to achieve a healthy, clear mind.

Revenge

Once you have finished working on regret, resentment, and rejection, then you can work on revenge. Entire nations are against one another because of the need for vengeance. We think of revenge and resentment not only to keep us safe, but to keep us on the Third Plane.

If we become so enlightened that we have virtuous feelings, we evolve and leave this plane of existence. When we have loved ones on this plane, we don't want to leave without them, so we reach for resentment, which will instantly bring us right back to the Third Plane. How many of us know that subconsciously we tend to be resentful and revengeful people? Left to its own devices, our undercurrent is really good at payback.

If someone cruelly rejects you, your undercurrent will look for ways to solve the problem. Once you do some belief work, you may find that your undercurrent is attempting to get revenge. Revenge can be a great motivator from time to time, as can the emotion of anger, both of which can delay enlightenment.

A good example of this was when I had my third child, Brandy. I had gained weight during pregnancy, and I was so angry with myself that I started to criticize myself. On top of that, my husband had a woman boss that kept him working double shifts when he didn't need to. Even as a young mother, I knew that she really liked him (in a sexual way). I thought: *One day I'm going to punch her in the nose. I'm only going to get one chance.*

This was the solution from my 20-year-old brain. So I started lifting weights, imagining hitting her in the nose. I exercised so much that I lost weight and looked so good that I didn't care if she took my husband, she could have him. I exercised my way back to health until I was releasing the right hormones. The motivation of revenge worked to my advantage, so sometimes these negative feelings can work for us in a good way, but I wasted a lot of time and energy, and I should have been motivated differently.

Revenge is an energy that keeps you going in circles instead of going forward. You can spend your whole life seeking some kind of justice for something that was wrongfully done to you. But is it really justice that you want, and are you going to spend a good part of your life in this endeavor?

There are two types of revenge: direct and subtle. For everyone that has hurt you in some way in your life, your undercurrent may be working toward revenge in a very subtle way. Your undercurrent will seek revenge in some situations, and the greatest revenge is success. But can you be a success without this kind of motivation? Your undercurrent can be satisfied if all those people who rejected you see your success. But it is better to be motivated through the higher self. Otherwise, you will never feel successful enough. If you are doing something such as healings because you love people, there will always be plenty. The key is to understand all aspects of your mind.

Once revenge, regret, resentment, and rejection are cleared, your ability to connect to the Creator will be enhanced.

BELIEF WORK FOR THE THREE Rs

Use the following exercises to help you work on issues with being rejected and the sorrow associated with it. First, find out what you regret, what you learned from it, and if you are finished learning from it. After you have done this, you can use the forgiveness exercise to forgive the person who caused the regret or work on self-forgiveness, and this may clear the need for revenge.

With yourself or with someone else, work on one resentment at a time, one instance of being rejected, and one regret for 30 minutes per person. Clearing revenge will be worked on last in a belief work session if it is needed.

To clear these issues, the reader or the practitioner must use the Creator throughout the exercise, with questions such as:

1.　'Creator, why do I have this regret?'

2.　'Creator, what did I learn from that?'

3.　'Have I learned all I need to from this situation? Do I have to keep it?'

Note: If the survival self, undercurrent self, and ego self are trying to keep a program associated with the regrets, resentments, or rejections, the client (or yourself) will respond to the questions about resentments or regrets with a dialogue similar to the one below:

Practitioner: 'What issue is bothering you?'

Client: 'No, I don't have any problems.'

Practitioner: 'What have you learned from any resentments or regrets?'

Client: 'I haven't learned anything from them.'

When working with yourself or with someone else, always go up to the Creator of All That Is for your answers, and they will be less combative.

Belief work example for resentment

Query: 'Who do you resent? Who hurt your feelings so long ago? What are you getting out of resenting this person?'

For more information, refer to the *Digging for Beliefs* book.

Belief work example for rejection

Query: 'Who rejected you? How do you feel about it? When did you feel rejected, and what did you learn from it? How did it motivate you? When did you reject another person?'

Undercurrent

Query: 'Are you getting even with this person or fixing it? What did you get out of being rejected? How did it motivate you?'

Belief work example for regret

When you are young, you make a lot of decisions, and this regret can keep you in the past; this is good to energy test for the following programs:

- 'I regret I didn't take my chance.'

- 'I regret that I hurt that person.'

- 'I regret how wild I was when I was younger.'

When you get older and more experienced, much of your regret goes away. You come to the realization that you were a young person, and harsh memories soften somewhat.

Note: The client should say why they have the regret and what they learned from it.

FORGIVENESS PRACTICE

A lack of forgiveness will block a connection to the Creator, so use the forgiveness exercise to complete the previous exercise of revenge, regret, resentment, and rejection for everyone that ever hurt your feelings. This can free your energy from someone that dislikes or hates you, someone that is sending you negative thoughts, someone that you hate or dislike, or someone that has done wrong to you in your life.

1. Go up to the Seventh Plane and connect to the Creator using the Road Map Meditation (see Introduction, page xiv).

2. Center yourself.

3. Begin by sending your consciousness down into the center of Mother Earth, into the energy of All That Is.

4. Bring the energy up through your feet, into your body, and through all the chakras.

5. Go up through your crown chakra, raise and project your consciousness out past the stars to the universe.

6. Go beyond the universe, through layers of light, through a golden light, past the jelly-like substance, which are the Laws, into a pearly, iridescent white light to the Seventh Plane of Existence.

7. Make the command or request, 'Creator of All That Is, it is commanded/requested that I forgive (name the person).

8. Imagine that the person who hurt you is standing in front of you.

9. Imagine telling this person how they have hurt you and what they have done to you.

10. Imagine that you tell the person who you forgive them for hurting you. As you tell this person who you forgive them, watch their reaction.

11. If the person is still standing in front of you in the vision, and they say that they are sorry, it means that they feel remorse on some level for what they have done.

12. If you come to the realization that they feel remorse for what they did, then the energy of forgiveness will protect you from angry thought forms that they send you. This also allows you to have compassion for them.

13. If, in the vision, they disappear into ash, this means that they have no remorse, and this takes away all negative thoughts from you.

14. This means that the hateful person will have to deal with their own negative thoughts, and they can no longer affect you.

15. What you have to learn from this person is done, and you are protected from them.

16. If they are still standing in front of you in the vision without saying anything and do not shrink, what you have to learn from this person is not finished.

17. This means that you have to do belief work about the situation. As you free yourself from the obligation of what they have to teach you, they will begin to get smaller and smaller in the vision.

18. Once finished, rinse yourself off with the Seventh Plane of Existence energy and stay connected to it.

Forgiveness is the strongest protection because when you say 'I forgive you' to someone, this means that you will no longer accept negative energy from them. In some instances, the person will apologize to you, and it may be that you can make amends. You should imagine doing this with only one person at a time. You can do this with more people as your skills improve, even with yourself.

STUCK IN THE PAST

One thing that regret and rejection can do is keep us stuck in the past from moving forward into the future because we replay regret and rejection over and over in our minds.

In one of my classes, I psychically watched my students go up to the Creator to remember their future. They didn't go forward in time as they were supposed to. They went off to this side or the other to remember what had happened to them. They didn't realize that the future is in front of them.

Then I realized that when they went up to look at their divine timing, they sat immobilized without any perception of where or what it was, without thinking that they had to look ahead into the future or back to the past. Your divine timing may have started five years ago when you began doing healings, or is still in the future.

RESETTING THE PAST, PRESENT, AND FUTURE

Some people are stuck in the past and have a difficult time making decisions. They don't know what actions will create the future. They come for healings and all they can talk about is the past. They say, 'I missed my chance, I was a quarterback, but I blew my knee out, my life is ruined.' Or 'I missed my chance. I started a business, but it failed, and my life is over.' These people are living in the past. To help them, don't get complicated, just refocus them by placing the memories of the past and the future in their proper context. This can help someone to move forward. The more connected we are to the higher self, the easier it is to move forward without the burdens of negative past experiences.

If you are doing belief work with another person (or yourself) and you hear them say, 'I'm stuck,' you should reply with, 'But if you weren't stuck, where would you be?' This will help to find out where the belief is coming from.

Some people go up to the Akashic records and see the 'end of the world.' What they are seeing is one of the many futures that can be changed because it is based on the choices that we make. Our civilization might go on for 10,000 years or for three more days, because we all have an influence on the future.

Downloads

The following downloads can help reset the mind:

'I know on every level that it is safe to realign my past, present, and future, and I am ready to move forward.'

'I know how to move forward with my life.'

'I can always learn from my past while moving into the future.'

'It is easy to remember my future.'

'It is easy to remember my past.'

To put the mind in the proper context, we do a 'reset' of the past, present, and future. In the exercise below, past experiences and events are organized into files as archives that can be accessed by the conscious mind, but the mind perceives them as past events that are behind, and the future events are in front of them. This clears the mind to move forward into the future.

If I was to look at my brain and I wanted to go back and look at my past, I would imagine the archives of the past directly behind my head traveling backward and the archives of the future in front of my forehead going forward.

If I go three years into the future, it is going to be more complex to perceive than it is three days. This is because the decisions of other people affect the outcome of the future through everyday interaction. There are, however, some things about the future that will not change.

Reset the Mind

This exercise helps with retention and organizing past information. I would use it with teenagers who are studying for a test, to help them go to the future where they could witness the test behind them, in the past. Then they could remember it, instead of looking all over their mind for the answers. You can use this exercise by yourself or with another person.

1.   Center yourself.

2.   Begin by sending your consciousness down into the center of Mother Earth, into the energy of All That Is.

3.   Bring the energy up through your feet, into your body, and bring the energy up through all the chakras.

4.   Go up through your crown chakra, raise and project your consciousness out past the stars to the universe.

5.   Go beyond the universe, through layers of light, through a golden light, past the jelly-like substance, which is the Laws, into a pearly, iridescent white light to the Seventh Plane of Existence.

6.   Make the command or request: 'Creator of All That Is, it is commanded/requested that a reset of all my memories be placed behind me in files, archives, or film strips as experiences that can be accessed as needed, and the future is in front of me as memory files leading into the

future that are easy for me to access. Witness as all past memories properly placed as archives behind me, and all future memories placed in front of me. Thank you! It is done, it is done, it is done.'

7.   When you are finished, go back to the tingly white light, say, 'It is done, it is done, it is done,' and open your eyes.

Once you have done this exercise, you may be able to see your past lives as archives. This is because the files go all the way back into your past genetic memories and into the future. This means that the archives of the future can be accessed by remembering the future and asking what happened the last time this happened.

THE BODY SPEAKS

As you become more psychically aware, you may hear the messages that the organs of the body send back and forth between them. Anytime an organ is out of balance, the messages sent out from it can be misunderstood.

Messages from microbes

Some of the messages that are making you confused might be from microbes in your own body. It is important to understand what are messages from the Creator and what are thought forms from the microscopic world that are created because of survival mode. Microbes only block you if you don't realize that they are influencing you.

Messages from candida

A little candida is a natural occurrence in the body, but when there is an imbalance, it can begin to get out of control. If you go on an alkaline diet to get rid of the overabundance of candida, the body has a craving for sugar. This craving comes from the candida broadcasting messages to the body for it to eat sugar. By the same token, if you go on a diet that excludes sugar and white flour, the candida will start to scream for sugar.

You will go through a conversation in your brain that tells you, 'I deserve it,' 'I can have it if I want it,' 'I cannot believe I am depriving myself of that candy bar because I want it.' 'I love myself enough to eat that candy bar.' This is why it is important to ask yourself where these cravings are coming from. I believe that it is possible to clear candida in the body by releasing resentment and guilt (since they go hand in hand). Remember that some cravings for food might mean that you need the nutrients that are in it, so it is always good to ask the Creator why you are having cravings.

Messages from bacteria

If someone psychic starts taking antibiotics for a bacterial infection, they may hear the message of 'This antibiotic is killing me. I going to quit taking it.' This isn't their own thoughts, but rather the bacteria that is being killed off by the antibiotic projecting itself onto the host.

Some bacteria in the body are beneficial, so it is only the negative bacteria that should be cleared. I believe that it is possible to clear bad bacteria in the body by releasing guilt.

Messages from parasites

Parasites send the host the same kinds of messages as bacteria when they are threatened. For instance, if someone uses medicine to kill a tapeworm, they all say the same thing two days into the treatment, 'This medicine is killing me.' This thought form is being projected from the tapeworm.

Messages from viruses

One of my students came to me and said her client was possessed, and no matter what she did to release it, it came back. Supposedly, they were possessed by a wayward She would say things like, 'They are possessed by entities.'

Since I knew that waywards don't usually possess people, I asked the Creator what she was seeing, and I was told she perceived viruses. I realized that the reader was intuitive enough and that viruses have thought forms and emit intelligence (of a kind), which could be mistaken as entities. So when the practitioner attempted to send the viruses to the light, they didn't listen.

What needs to be done with viruses is belief work to change them to a harmless state. It wasn't that this Thetahealer was overly superstitious. I knew what viruses looked and felt like after thousands of readings. But how do you teach someone else to know the difference in identifying them?

Simple, you go up to the Creator and ask, 'Creator, what is this? Is it a virus?'

Sometimes, when you work with clients, you will be talking to their sickness rather than the person. Once you understand the difference between talking to the client or their disease, they will be a lot happier with the session.

If you start working with people who have viruses such as HIV, you should know that it may tell the host things like, 'You need me,' 'I helped you change your life,' 'Without me, you will go back to what you were before' and 'I am helping you.' These are the projected thoughts of the virus toward the host.

If you have a virus that is making you sick, sometimes the thought that is projected is: 'I'm a healer. I can't be sick, I'm a terrible healer, I should just quit.'

Toxins

Exposure to toxins such as petroleum-based products, chemicals, heavy metals such as arsenic, mercury, lead, cadmium, chromium, nickel, and manganese can make it difficult to understand the highest answers because they create negative emotions. When these toxins are cleared from the body, it will be much easier to connect to the highest truth.

The thoughts of others

Some people are very intuitive and sometimes don't know the difference between their thoughts and others'. Getting to know the pure essence of the Creator will get them to realize the difference between their thoughts and those of others. When you are a child, it is easy to know the difference between these energies because you are connected to the Creator.

We perceive thought forms from all kinds of things: inanimate objects that we touch, other people's thoughts, especially those of people who are close to us, and we are being pounded by radio waves from cell phones.

THE DNA FIGHT FOR SUPREMACY

Our DNA is so programmed to survive that we have to fight the genetic ego that tells us, 'we are better than others.' There is likely going to be someone in your genetic line that believed that their people are the only 'chosen ones.' This thought form blocks you from getting clear answers if these beliefs are not changed. To the Creator, we are all 'chosen.'

You may hear messages that tell you that 'There is only one like you,' 'You are the one,' 'You are better,' and so on, but these messages are *not* the Creator. If you hear these kinds of messages, it is important to explore whether you have any beliefs of superiority or prejudice against others.

It is worth noting that most of your DNA programs are positive in nature. Our ancestors learned many virtues and beneficial survival instincts that have been handed down to us. Sometimes, we only need to understand our genetic beliefs, not change all of them.

HEALER FATIGUE

Most healers tend to have workaholic tendencies and often have to work two jobs to support their healing business, or they have a healing business and work until they exhaust their adrenals.

When you have a program that you cannot stop working, your adrenals become stressed, and the temper becomes short. Many healers will tell me that they need to keep better control of their temper, but it more likely they are using it just to get through life. They get up in the morning already tired, and to keep going, they raise their cortisol levels, so they get angry.

Being overtired causes anger that causes fear, and that blocks clear messages. It may have nothing to do with how 'spiritual' someone is, it has to do with exhaustion. And I have to tell you, healers don't quit until they can't get up anymore. It's like, 'hardwired' into them, so knowing when to rest and take care of our little house of the soul is super important. Your body is your house on this plane, and without it, we don't get to play!

EXHAUSTION

Some healers have type-A personalities and tend to take on as many clients as they can. This can exhaust someone pretty fast. The Creator can give you energy, but not if the only way that you can rest is if you work until you are exhausted as an excuse to rest. The undercurrent loves to use exhaustion as an excuse to rest, so it is important to do some belief work. Telling yourself that you will rest doesn't mean you will actually do it. And what does rest mean to you? Does rest mean seeing the sights on your day off? You may need a vacation from your days off! Learning how to rest and actually doing it is very important.

Exhaustion can block you from getting all the right answers, but not completely. You may have to go up to the Creator and keep saying 'my highest truth,' and you will free yourself from the fetters of the mind. If you are exhausted, and you go up and ask, 'What is wrong with me?' The answer is going to be, 'You are exhausted.'

FEAR

Fear is a natural survival response. But the wrong kind of fear blocks clear messages. This can happen when a client has a health challenge and is asking for advice. When a client tells you something like 'You have to help me, you are my last hope,' the practitioner must set aside their fear of failure. Remember, the client only needs 30 seconds without fear for healing to happen. If you are afraid to ask for clear messages from the Creator, or if you have a lot of fear in giving a reading, then this needs to be cleared for good communication.

ANGER

Learning how to heal without being angry is very important. Let's say you do a healing on a client, and it doesn't work. You see the client suffering and get angry at the Creator. This is a genetic belief but can also be a habit.

In this case, act as though when you are doing belief work – as though you are a private detective who is solving the case. Or act as though you are a scientist. You did a healing but it didn't work, so try a new formula. If you use these approaches, you won't become angry with the Creator. God doesn't make people get sick because, in most instances, it takes a while for someone to get sick.

Anger can block us from the highest truth. If you are getting an answer when angry, common sense is huge. It may not be the highest truth. If you are angry and decide to do a reading and go up for the highest answer, leave the anger behind because it makes your thoughts heavy.

Some people don't realize when they are angry, deep down, perhaps because they were never allowed to be angry. But the subconscious knows when you are angry. If you are in the middle of a fight with your spouse and you want to go up to the Creator and ask advice, you must realize you will not be angry when you get to the Creator. The fight will be over, and you will forget why you are angry. If you want to stay angry, you won't as long as you are connected to the Creator.

If you have an angry, heated conversation with yourself while driving and you tell yourself: 'I should just leave home,' and then you go up to the Creator and ask if you should leave, you are going to forget why you wanted to leave home. The Creator will say things like 'Breathe, just breathe. It's okay.'

ME, ME, ME – GIVE ME, MINE, I WANT...

These are some of the traits to watch for in yourself and in others because they can all block clear communication with the Creator:

• An exaggerated sense of self-importance

• Preoccupation with fantasies of unlimited success, power, brilliance, beauty, or ideal love

- Belief in being 'special' and only understood by, or should associate with, people (or institutions) who are also 'special' or of high status

- Requires excessive admiration

- Has a sense of self-entitlement

- Is interpersonally exploitative

- Lacks empathy

- Is often *envious* of others or believes others are *envious* of him or her

- Has arrogant, haughty behaviors or attitudes

Are you aware of the feelings of others, or are you obtuse? Do you impose yourself upon others regardless of their feelings? To be a good Thetahealers, we have to know what is going on in someone else's paradigm. By the same token, we need to keep our space clean. We need to live our lives and not go out of our way to intentionally hurt someone. But we also need to understand that we can defend our right to be, and to be able to keep things in order in our lives. We should also have a moral compass of what is right and wrong.

If you are immersed in mine, mine, mine, give me, give me, give me, I want... it is difficult to reach the Creator or be a good healer. Manifesting good things into your life isn't being narcissistic. Don't get me wrong, you can manifest anything for yourself, but if the only thing you think or care about is yourself, it will block you from getting clear messages. This is why some healers have pets, girlfriends (or boyfriends), clients, brothers, sisters, mothers, and fathers that they spend a lot of time helping to keep them from being completely self-absorbed.

BLAMING THE CREATOR

If you blame the Creator for something difficult that is going on in your life, this blocks you from reaching the Seventh Plane. This is mostly from a genetic program that the Creator is doing something to us and is centered around pain and fear of death. It is important to realize how ridiculous it is to blame the Creator for the gift of life.

GIVING THE CREATOR ULTIMATUMS

Ultimatums to the Creator are all in the mind. If you obsess with thoughts such as, 'Creator, if you give me a new car I will heal people,' or 'If you don't heal this person I won't believe in you anymore,' it means you are talking to your subconscious and not reaching the Creator. The energy of creation doesn't have to prove anything to someone. Giving ultimatums to the Creator makes it impossible to reach the Creator because they are such heavy thought forms. Ultimatums are the creation of one of the first three aspects, and you are simply stuck in your mind.

You can say things such as, 'Creator, I'm going to follow my path, please protect my children when I'm working.' This is not an ultimatum.

People come to me and say, 'If you heal me, I will dedicate my life to God.' Well, it is the Creator that is going to heal them! They do not have to bargain with the Creator, or with me.

In ancient times it was common for people to bargain with the Creator. They would go up to the Fifth Plane and say: 'Creator, if you heal this person, I will give my right arm for them. If you don't heal this person, I'm not going to believe in you anymore. If you don't show me a sign tomorrow, I am done with you.'

This kind of scenario doesn't work because the energy of creation is a living force, and you are alive because of it. It doesn't have to prove to you that it exists when it is the basis of everything. Similarly, I have had students say, 'If this pencil moves, I know ThetaHealing is true,' and the pencil moved!

Ultimatums are the brain's way of not having to move something. You don't go up to the Creator and say, 'Creator, I'm not going to finish my life path unless you do this for me.'

PEER PRESSURE

Sometimes we might do things to please others not because we want to but due to peer pressure. Any time we are in this way, it is going to block us from getting messages. It is important to recognize when this is happening.

When I tell people about some of my healings, they sometimes say, 'Prove it.' When I teach the DNA 3 class, I have people move a pencil or a tissue with their mind. When someone challenges you and says, 'You do it,' the brain can freeze up. This is a lot of peer pressure. But if you go up to someone and say, 'Let me help you do it,' it works. This takes the pressure off you.

Of course, when people say, 'You are a healer, heal it,' this too is a lot of peer pressure. After all, the Creator is the healer. The thing is, if someone challenges you to 'prove it,' they wouldn't believe it if you proved it to them. Clear your beliefs, and quit worrying about what others think about you.

I have had several Thetahealers try to prove they are abundant. They would purchase all kinds of stuff, so the other practitioners and teachers would think they were abundant. But really, they just got in debt that overwhelmed them.

Downloads

Use the following downloads to help keep clear channels of communication with the Creator.

- 'I know what it feels like for my family to know I am following my heart.'

- 'I know what it feels like to be a successful healer.'

- 'I know how to work with others as friends.'

BRAIN CANDY

When you start to go up to the Creator, your brain opens in certain ways, and you can get a lot of psychic information from many sources that I call brain candy. Don't get me wrong, I like some kinds of brain candy, such as infrared saunas and colored light therapy which are powered by the Laws of the universe. But you can get caught up in information that keeps your mind over-occupied, constantly looking for more theories and conspiracies. This can be anything that isn't the pure knowledge of the Creator. Brain candy can also be all those little truths that are true (or mainly true) and can obsessively occupy the mind for long periods, so much so that it interferes with our connection to the Creator.

How do you get out of the brain candy when your brain is designed to explore new things? You won't get away from it, not completely, but you can minimize energies that do not serve you. The human brain is run by chemicals and neurotransmitters that must be in balance. The brain becomes balanced when you go up to the Creator. The more you go up to the Creator, the more you see your life from the Creator's perspective. From the Creator's perspective, everything is easy. When I stop and look at every decision that I am making, I realize that there is a purpose to it all, and I am finally at peace.

The more you open up, the more you may come to many realizations. You may find out that your religion is cool or not so cool. You may get information from the far reaches of the universe about the multitude of races living in other star systems. You may hear that you are a star seed from a far galaxy.

It doesn't matter if you are a star seed and have connected to some consciousness from the Pleiades, Arcturus, or Orion. The chances of this planet being seeded from outside influences are very likely but don't get caught up in this brain candy.

You can get so much information when your mind is open in theta that you forget what is important: a connection to *one energy*. What is important is to remember your abilities, change limiting beliefs, and help your family line, those who are on the Fourth Plane, and those who are here.

We should be aware of all the planes of existence without being so caught up in the brain candy that can be associated with them. Brain candy is often good, but we should never forget the truth: we connect to the Creator first.

●●●

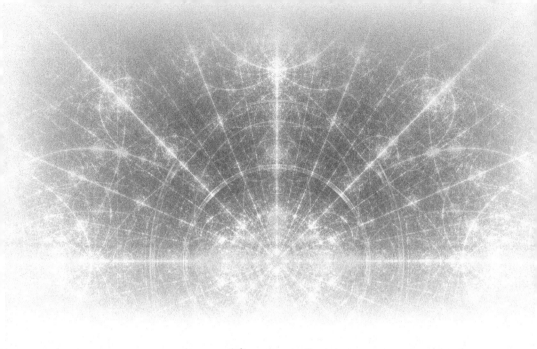

Chapter 8

PRINCIPLES FOR
CLEAR MESSAGES

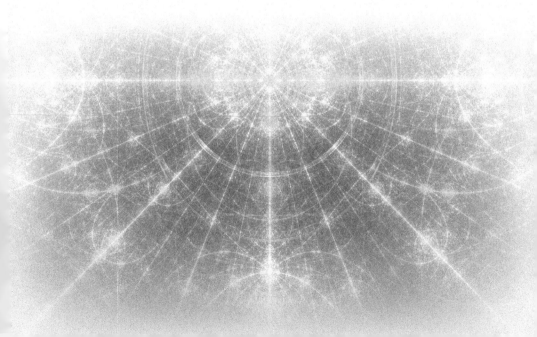

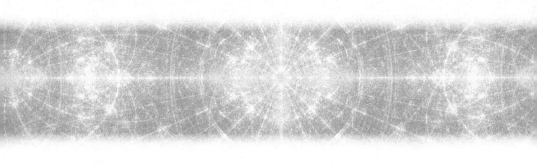

In the previous chapter, we covered some topics that block us from connecting to the highest energy. This chapter defines the principles that make connecting to the Creator much easier.

SPIRITUAL COMMON SENSE

The Creator's energy is such that it will not accept negative requests. For instance, the Law of Free Agency, the Creator, will not give your boss a heart attack because you don't like him or her.

What is the Creator to you, and what kinds of messages would you get from this pure energy? Would the Creator be negative or dualistic? Never! Would the Creator tell you to jump off a cliff? Never! You must ask, 'Is this the highest answer?' Always use logic with psychic intuition and ask for the highest truth and keep asking until you *know* it is.

Once you are given advice from the Creator, you have to follow through with it and put it into action. The mind can create all kinds of reasons not to follow through with the pure message. Remember to have faith in the intelligent, knowing the love of the Creator.

INTERPRETATION

When you channel pure information, the messages you receive from the Creator must be interpreted correctly. Even information from pure channeling can be misinterpreted by the ego or the undercurrent. If you do not understand a message, ask more questions until you do.

You should not believe any channeled book until you have asked the Creator about its content. History books are the same. The knowledge of history is filtered through many different influences and is not necessarily what really happened. This includes what is posted on the internet and some media stations. These streams of information are only as good as what is motivating the people behind them, who often have a curious lack of a moral compass. When you read something, ask, 'Creator, what is the real motivation behind this information?' Always ask for pure information.

ACCOMPLISH

One thing that can help make a better connection is to have an idea of what you can accomplish. Go up to the Creator and ask to be shown three things that you can accomplish, and you will be amazed.

The Creator can do anything. Nothing is more powerful than the Creator, but as you work on your beliefs, your level of witnessing can change. The more you practice your abilities, the more you trust, the more confirmation you get, the more you learn, and the more you can do. Do not block all you may accomplish.

The fact is that most Thetahealers try harder, and they don't give up until they connect with the Creator. This is the formula for success.

MOTIVATION

One of the fears Thetahealers often express is not being able to help someone and that the healing won't work. But when they move the fear out of the way for just a few seconds, then healings can happen. However, the healer must be perceptive enough to know if the fear is theirs or the client's. When a healer connects to a client, they also connect to the fears of their family or spouse. Always go up and ask, 'Creator, where are these feelings coming from?'

If your motivation is loving and helping others, you are going to do a lot better with abundance. If your motivation is from fear, you may not do as well. The way that this works is as follows: Your higher self knows your divine timing: your life purpose of being a healer. You know on some level that you are going to be a healer. The Creator will make sure that you have bills to pay so that you have to go to work to pay your bills to keep you being a healer. You have to go to work on Friday because you have to pay the electric bill. You have to go to work on Thursday because you have to pay the doctor's bill.

These are all great motivations, but money is just paper. So, you can either pay a $50 bill or a $50,000 bill, and you will still be able to make it as long as you keep being a healer. Wouldn't it be good if you programmed yourself that you were doing it out of love instead of just for the electric bill?

I'm not saying that finances are people's only motivation, but if you make a commitment with yourself that you will help others, your money problems will become fewer.

DEVELOP VIRTUES

The soul is working toward virtues, and they are its main objective. It creates situations in someone's life to develop them. The more you work on and achieve virtues, the clearer your answers. Get up every morning, thankful that you are alive and your body is doing a good job. Thank the Creator for everything in your life. Go up to the Creator and ask what virtues you need to master.

THE RIGHT QUESTION

Years ago, I had a student call me in tears telling me that his passport had expired and they wouldn't let them on the plane.

He didn't tell me where he was going, so I went up and looked to the future and told him, 'You know, you don't want to go to Bali right now.' He calmed down a little and went home from the airport.

That night, there was a terrorist bomb attack in Bali. The student called me the next morning and said, 'How did you know that? How did you know I was going to Bali?'

I told him. 'Because I went up and *asked the right question*: "Creator, is there a reason this person is not able to travel?"'

The Creator told me, 'Avoid travel to Bali. Because he cannot travel, he is safe.'

THE LIFE-FORCE

We are teaching people to go up and connect to the Creator. But we have to bring people to the awareness that they are already connected to the life-force. We are alive because of the life-force. As we change beliefs, we will eventually feel the tingly energy of the life-force.

UNSEEN FORCES

One thing that helps to connect with the Creator and use the life-force is to realize and accept that there are unseen forces around you. If you accept that they are around you, things are much easier. An important ThetaHealing question is: 'Am I crazy?'

Wait for your higher self to say, 'You are okay.' Always tell yourself you are okay.

Get used to the unseen forces. If you encounter a wayward spirit that bothers you, send it to the light. Doors will open by themselves, and miracles will happen. Just relax, you've *got* this!

BRAVERY

It is hard to live without fear if you keep begging the Creator for courage. If you ask for courage, you will also get the fear that comes with it. Courage is facing your fears, overcoming them is bravery. It takes a brave person to admit they have fears. Change your request to the Creator and ask for bravery. Bravery is having no fear and recognizing all the times you've had courage.

Realize that some things are not about calmness or fear. They just are what they are. If you get nervous in some situations, this is normal. The day you have no emotions is the time you should not be a reader or a healer. Remember how amazing you are. You must have courage and bravery to be different from others.

TRUE DISCERNMENT

True discernment of what is right and what is wrong comes with time and experience. You have to know how to make the right moral choice. If you get a message and it doesn't sound morally right, then it isn't.

REFOCUSING THOUGHTS

If your mind starts to wander and you become unfocused, your connection to the Seventh Plane can be lost. Refocus your thoughts. If this happens and you get a message, ask yourself, is this a message that comes from the Creator?

One thing that helps is to write down what you want to accomplish and manifest, but allow yourself to focus and refocus your thoughts as the future changes. As the future becomes the present, things might change or grow in a different way than you intended. This is when you have to refocus your thoughts to this alteration in your manifestation.

HELPING OTHERS

If you are bothered by what other people think of you, there is a secret you should know. When you help others, your self-esteem grows in the right way, and it is really easy to connect to the Creator.

TRUST YOUR DECISIONS

Another important point is to trust your decisions. Say to yourself, 'I made this decision. What good things happened because of it?'

One of the most important things that you can do is to look back over all your decisions and ask the Creator why you made them. You will discover that you made decisions for amazing reasons that brought you to who you are now. Look at every decision that you make, and you will discover how your inner aspects are working for you and against you. Once you see how they are working for you, your ability to manifest will be improved.

TRUST THE CREATOR

Life takes some strange turns. When I took nuclear security training, I didn't realize it would prepare me for what I do today. It gave me a chance to do sketches and readings on breaks. It also showed me the world could be both good and bad. It put me in the right place to learn about naturopathic medicine, but this wasn't my first decision. My first decision was to become a geologist and study volcanoes, but instead, I made another decision based on trusting the Creator. This trust helped me to be prepared to learn about my environment, to travel, and to understand people.

For a healer to be the best they can be, there must be a good relationship with the Creator. The best way to have this is to learn how to trust the Creator.

DIVINE TIMING

Remember, divine timing is your path, your purpose, and when the universe is there to support you, the timing is right. With free agency, we created a plan before we came to this planet with a purpose.

One thing that can stop you from being able to see your divine timing is the survival part of your brain. This is because the survival part of you is afraid you will leave your family behind. Divine timing is a very cool thing. Do you know that you can bring your family with you on your divine-timing path, so they can be enlightened too?

If you can see your divine timing, you can do some very cool things. Instead of surviving, you can start living and become happy. If you are on your divine path, you can become physically strong. If you know what your divine path is, you can create the reality you want. You can recognize that you are trying to fix something from the past.

DIVINE INTERVENTION

Divine intervention is when divine timing comes into play and pushes you to your path and continues to push you forward. You have a divine path, and you came here for a reason, sometimes with two or three paths to complete. I remember looking at my divine timing when I was in my 30s, and I saw myself talking in front of groups of people. I remember thinking, 'That isn't like me, how could this be?' But when I started doing readings and teaching small classes, it was natural and easy.

MEDITATION

You might be blocking your divine timing, so it is useful to know that divine intervention is working in your life. This exercise will show you all the different times that divine intervention has come into your life. Allow this knowledge to reset your mind in the same way as if you had reorganized the past, present, and future.

1. Take a deep breath in and close your eyes.

2. Imagine energy coming up through the bottom of your feet, moving up to the top of your head, making a beautiful ball of light.

3. Pretend that you are in that ball of light.

4. I want you to imagine that you are going up past the universe, through layers and layers of light, through a golden light, through a thick jelly-like substance, into a tingly white light that is the Seventh Plane of Existence.

5. Make the command/request, 'Creator of All That Is, it is commanded/requested to show me my next divine intervention now. Thank you. It is done, it is done, it is done.'

6. Go into the future to see the next divine intervention.

7. When you are finished, come back to this time through the tingly white light and take a deep breath in.

If you didn't see your divine timing, it might be one of five things:

1. Go up to the Creator and ask for anything that is blocking you from allowing you to achieve your divine timing.

2. Go up to the Creator and ask, 'What am I missing?' If you don't get an immediate answer, ask again.

3. You might be afraid of your divine timing.

4. You saw your divine timing but didn't understand it.

5. You are already doing your divine timing.

BRING THE FAMILY TO ENLIGHTENMENT

Every soul knows that if you have an awakening of enlightenment too quickly, you may get bored and not want to stay on

Earth. So many of us are homesick for the full energy of the Fifth Plane. This is why it is important to bring the energy of love from the Fifth Plane to Earth and let it spread into the family.

Many people are afraid to become enlightened or ascended because they do not want to leave their families behind. This fear comes from the undercurrent part of us. But what if your family became enlightened along with you? It does not have to be only you that moves toward enlightenment, but your family can as well. Changing to the right beliefs can positively affect your family and help them evolve.

Many healers have the belief that they cannot teach their family members to become enlightened, but this is not true. They get stuck with the idea that their children will always be children or that their teenagers will always be teenagers. But children grow up and evolve. When they are older, their perceptions change. The family needs to know that your belief systems of spirituality are not a threat to them.

LIVING

Project love to the world and focus on living a life that your soul is proud of. The more that you live your life this way, the clearer your answers from the Creator will be. Don't wait until next month or next year to realize you are happy today.

THE BATTLE WITH THE SURVIVAL SELF

Being consciously aware of the survival self will help with enlightenment because you will realize when you are doing something from a survival instinct. Realization of needless reactions from the survival self will help you to live life to the full.

It is very important to be kind to your body with your thoughts. If we get up in the morning and say, 'My body is no good,' 'I'm too fat,' or 'I'm too skinny,' the body might accept these thoughts as a reality. Some positive programs that serve me well are, 'I have a resilient body' and 'Teaching ThetaHealing and connecting to the Creator gives me physical strength.'

One thing to avoid is to allow psychic abilities to develop before the mind and body have proper discernment to handle them. If the human body cannot keep up with the growth of psychic abilities there may be a crash, so it is best to take things a step at a time. The only way to avoid this is to start sorting out your thoughts. The more virtuous thoughts, the stronger the body. In one way physical exercise is good, but exercising virtue is better. The more virtuous the thoughts, the more the body will shift and change with the growth of the soul. The more negative thoughts we have, the more stagnant and attached to the earth we become. Because of too many negative thoughts, a battle begins inside us.

The battle is between the old self and the new self that is forming with the virtuous thoughts. As you become more enlightened, the more you may fear to lose your old identity. All of this fear is from the survival self trying to keep us in our body on this Third Plane. This comes from an ancient belief system that is instinctual in many of us.

Put simply, this belief system is as follows: If you attain and maintain a higher thought-form vibration, you would want to go to other dimensions and leave the mortal body. If you could be in another place of pure love where everyone treated one another with love and respect, would you want to stay on this earth? This is why my students say things like, 'I know I am not getting where I want to be.' They are Ascended Masters that are waking up and instinctively, they know there is so much more to their existence. These new feelings can be perceived as a threat to the physical body by the survival self.

The Creator tells me this battle is a waste of time. If we could have more virtuous thoughts, our body would be healthy, and the survival self would not feel threatened. Now we can be ascended in a human body and help the world ascend. Everyone goes through the battle between the survival self and the higher self. If they have not gone through it, they will. This is why it is important to consciously sort out what our brain and survival self are doing, so it is the higher self that directs our life from every experience it is learning. Sort out your thoughts and reprogram your survival self so that it can be healthy and move forward.

ILLNESS

Illness can make it difficult for someone to get clear answers from the Creator because the survival self is on high alert. But as long as someone can imagine going up to the Seventh Plane, healing can still happen if they are persistent.

Some healers would rather be around sick people because, for the most part, they are at least polite and nice. The healer needs to understand that when someone becomes well, their personality might change. I can't tell you how many people I know who were awesome when they were sick and became difficult when they became well, but sometimes this works the opposite way.

DETOXING – THOUGHTS AND THE PHYSICAL BODY

One thing that can help the ability to meditate for clear answers is detoxing your body. I'm not telling you that you cannot get the highest answer if your body is toxic, and you don't feel well. I have known people who were close to death that got clear answers. But if your body is toxic, it can be distracting enough to make it difficult to get up to your crown and maintain the right kind of concentration.

This is why detoxing your body with gentle cleanses, regular exercise, and a good diet can be beneficial. However, detoxing with cleanses are not for everyone. Doing a physical detox takes a lot of physical strength. Many people take all kinds of detoxes to clean the organs, but detoxing your thoughts is the best way to detox your body.

READINGS MAKE YOU NICER

You are much nicer on the days that you do readings because when you help people, the brain releases the chemical serotonin. When I can, I do a reading in the morning to put myself in the right frame of mind for the day. If you go two or three days without connecting to the Seventh Plane, the highest truth is more elusive. But if you get up every morning and connect to the Seventh Plane, it makes it much easier to get clear answers.

LEAVE PAIN BEHIND

One thing that helps to get clear answers is being able to live without pain. Living with pain can be a great teacher, but living without pain is much better. If you are in constant pain, it is still possible to connect to the Creator, and it doesn't necessarily keep you from getting clear messages, but it can be a challenge. It is a lot easier to be psychic when you leave the pain behind. Think of how clear you can be *without* pain.

Many healers seem to have a difficult time accepting help from others, so it is good to explore why this is with belief work. They are very good at relieving pain in others but not their own. I know of healers that are working with numerous clients and teaching classes that simply deal with their pain and still go forward.

I think pain is one thing that keeps them on this planet. As long as they are in pain, they can still connect on the same level as everyone else. If they were out of pain, their abilities would magnify faster, and they might be afraid of the next step that has something to do with their undercurrent. If they took the next step, they would not be in pain.

I have a theory about pain. I think that if we work on our undercurrent, we will find out what we are getting out of the pain, then we can live without it.

ASK THE CREATOR FOR THE ISSUE AND WHAT IS BLOCKING YOU

Go up to the Creator to ask for answers about the motivations of the survival self, the ego, and the undercurrent. Ask the Creator 'is it the survival self, the ego, the undercurrent, the higher self, or the Creator?' What is the undercurrent self doing? Where did it begin? Is it the ego self? What is the higher-self learning?

Optional: Go to the Creator to find the bottom beliefs and undercurrent motivations with yourself or with a partner.

Downloads

Use the following downloads to help clear problems and issues:

'I know what it feels like to clear problems in minutes.'

'I know what it feels like to know I am important and a spark of God.'

'I know what it feels like to live my life without always being in pain.'

'I know how and what it feels like to clear enough beliefs so that I can keep up with my abilities.'

'I know how and what it feels like to make a difference.'

MESSAGES FROM THE PLANES

Each of the **Seven Planes of Existence** has an energy signature, a feeling of its own. This is why it is important to ask:

- 'What does a message from each plane sounds like?'

- 'What does it feel like?'

- 'Where is it coming from?'

- 'Who or what is it that is giving the message?'

- 'What is it saying to you?'

- 'What are the energies inherent in each of the planes?'

For example, on the Fifth Plane, there are masters like Christ, the angels, your heavenly father and mother that all have a distinctive energy. When you become more experienced, you will be able to know the difference between the 'All That Is' energy and the Fifth Plane masters.

Some people will only accept a healing from the energy of a specific plane of existence, and to witness the healing, you have to know the energy of the Plane. There may be times when you go up to the Creator and request a healing, and you may get the message: 'Because of their belief system, this person will only accept a healing from the Fifth Plane.' When this happens, it isn't uncommon to see an angel from the Fifth Plane in the healing.

If you ask the Sixth Plane Laws a question such as, 'What do I need for my body to feel better?' The answer might be, 'You need to lie under green light,' or 'Eat better, get more sleep, and quit messing around at night.' This kind of message is likely from a Law. But if you go up and ask the Creator, you might hear, 'Oh, you have a wonderful body. It tries so hard. Just love your body.'

To bend the energy of the Sixth Plane Laws, you must master enough virtues. This is because virtues are lite-thought forms

143

so powerful that they can move across the universe faster than the speed of light. Negative thought forms are heavy and never leave the earth. With the right combination of virtues, some Laws can be bent to create change, and as a high Fifth Plane being, you may remember how to work with them.

A good example of the way these messages from the planes are different comes from the time when a man came up to me in class and said, 'Vianna, that lady over there gave me a reading and told me that I am cheating on my wife.'

Well, I could see that this was true. He *was* cheating on his wife. If I were to go up and give him a Fourth Plane answer, it would be about sacrifice, suffering, dualism, or an initiation of some kind. For example: 'You are cheating on your wife. You should be ashamed of yourself. There are a lot of people who you are hurting. You will have to work very hard to make this right.'

If I were to go up and I give him a Fifth Plane answer, it would be dualistic: 'Why are you cheating on your wife?'

The Sixth Plane answer would be: 'It is true.'

But if you go up and ask the Creator, the Seventh Plane response is softer and would be: 'It must be hard to love two people.' This message doesn't support cheating, it just means the energy of creation knows this man. It knows what is in his heart and that everyone is different, and he may want to explore the possibility that he is afraid to love anyone completely.

You can only work with the Laws if you have mastered enough virtues. Because virtues are thoughts that are lite, thoughts such as resentment are heavy. The thought form of virtues is powerful. They can move across the universe faster than the speed of light. With the right combination of virtues, you can remember how to bend some Laws to create change.

THE FEELING OF THE SEVEN PLANES OF EXISTENCE

The following exercises will help you to know the difference between the planes of existence. During a belief work session, it is important to be able to discern where the message is coming from. It also makes you aware of yourself and where your messages are coming from and to know how to reach the highest truth.

Ask yourself: 'What would it feel like if you were in the energy of pure love talking to the highest intelligence?' Sometimes we might go to the Seventh Plane and then end up answering a question from the Sixth Plane. What is important is to know *what* you are doing and *where* you are connecting to.

If you are working with another person, have them take you up to the Seventh Plane, make the command/request to ask for the Fourth, Fifth, Sixth, and Seventh Plane answer to the question. If you are working with yourself, go up to the Seventh Plane to make the command/request for the answer to the question, then go to the chosen plane of existence.

The person having the reading will think of a question that they will ask the reader. This question should be a serious question and is the same question for each of the planes.

In this exercise, we don't go to the First or Second Planes. This is because an answer from the First Plane crystals would come incredibly slowly. If you asked the trees of the Second Plane if you should get a divorce, they would ask you, 'what is a divorce?' The answer from the Second Plane fairy kingdom might be 'Yay! Oh boy! What is divorce?'

FEELING THE PLANES

In this exercise, go up to the Seventh Plane and then to one of the planes of existence.

1. Take a deep breath in. Center yourself.

2. Imagine energy coming up through the bottoms of your feet, going up through the top of your head in a ball of light, imagine you are in that ball of light, go up past the universe through layers of light, through a golden light,

through a thick jelly-like substance, and into a tingly, white-white light.

3. Make the request/command: 'Creator of All That Is, it is requested/commanded a Fourth Plane answer to this person's question. Thank you. It is done, it is done, it is done.'

4. Imagine going to the Fourth Plane to wait for the answer. The reader will go to the Fourth Plane to ask for an answer to the client's question.

5. The reader will indicate to the client that they are ready to answer their question from the perspective of the Fourth Plane. This may have something to do with sacrifice or initiation.

6. Make sure they go up to the tingly white light when they are finished.

GO TO THE SEVENTH PLANE TO THE FIFTH PLANE

1. Take a deep breath in. Center yourself.

2. Imagine energy coming up through the bottoms of your feet, going up through the top of your head in a ball of light, imagine you are in that ball of light, go up past the universe through layers of light, through a golden light,

through a thick jelly-like substance, and into a tingly, white-white light.

3.   Make the request/command: 'Creator of All That Is, it is requested/commanded a Fifth Plane answer to this person question. Thank you. It is done, it is done it, is done.'

4.   Imagine going to the Fifth Plane to wait for the answer.

5.   The reader will go to the Fifth Plane to ask an answer to the question.

6.   The reader will indicate to the client that they are ready. This answer may have a little bit of dualism. Make sure they go up to the tingly white light when they are finished.

GO TO THE SEVENTH PLANE TO THE SIXTH PLANE

1.   Take a deep breath in. Center yourself.

2.   Imagine energy coming up through the bottoms of your feet, going up through the top of your head in a ball of light, imagine you are in that ball of light, go up past the universe through layers of light, through a golden light, through a thick jelly-like substance, and into a tingly, white-white light.

3.   Make the request/command: 'Creator of All That Is, it is requested/commanded a Sixth Plane answer to this

person's question. Thank you. It is done, it is done, it is done.'

4.   Imagine going to the Fifth Plane to wait for the answer.

5.   The reader will go to the Sixth Plane and ask for an answer to the question.

6.   The reader will indicate to the client that they are ready. The answer will likely be the raw truth. Make sure they go up to the tingly white light when they are finished.

GUIDE TO THE SEVENTH PLANE

1.   Take a deep breath in. Center yourself.

2.   Imagine energy coming up through the bottoms of your feet, going up through the top of your head in a ball of light, imagine you are in that ball of light, go up past the universe through layers of light, through a golden light, through a thick jelly-like substance, and into a tingly, white-white light.

3.   Make the request/command: 'Creator of All That Is, it is requested/commanded a Seventh Plane answer to this person's question. Thank you. It is done, it is done, it is done.'

4.   Imagine going to the Seventh Plane to wait for the answer.

5.   The reader will go to the Seventh Plane and ask for an answer. The reader will indicate to the client that they are ready to answer the question. The answer will come from the most intelligent, loving energy ever created.

6.   Make sure they go up to the tingly white light when they are finished.

EVOLUTION OF THE FAMILY LINE

The DNA of the family line is incredibly powerful. The instinct to ensure that the family line continues can be such a distraction that it can stop you from getting clear messages from the Creator. Thetahealers seem to take this responsibility on to themselves, as there is always one person in a family that has more negative genetic beliefs that need to be altered. The person who has the most genetic beliefs to alter is the 'messiest' in the family. They are sometimes hoarders and have a lot of stuff. If someone has many genetic beliefs that need altering, they might begin to gain weight for no reason. If this happens to you and your house gets messy, clearing the clutter and watch the beliefs that come up. The same will happen if you gain weight and then begin to lose it.

Some people have 30-year-old children that are still not grown up yet, and others are taking care of their elderly parents.

When the people in your family line evolve, you may become so focused on these family members that you forget all else. You may even be dealing with messages from your own DNA that tell you things like: 'Everyone in my family failed, but I will succeed.' Now that the people in your genetic line know that you are changing your genetic beliefs, they likely have a list of their own, but it is best to go up to the Creator and ask what needs to be changed.

So now, with the ability to identify your thoughts on an aspect level, you may understand yourself better. Knowing the difference between the aspects – survival, undercurrent, ego, and higher self – allows you to be consciously aware and focus on your purpose. Now you know how to determine if your answers are from the most intelligent, loving truth.

•••

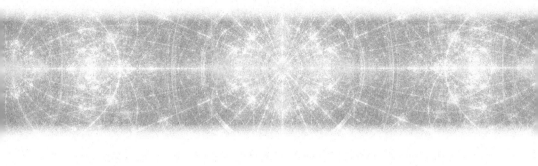

FINAL MESSAGES
FROM VIANNA

Talk to the Creator every day; thank the Creator every day and honor life in all its forms. Slow down and notice the air and the light. Appreciate life.

Go up and ask the Creator so you can avoid having to learn the hard way.

All is not what it seems

Thoughts move faster than light; they move and have essence, so be careful what you think.

So much of our time is wasted upon useless thought forms. We must learn to focus and direct our thought-energy to the divine consciousness.

Do something to be proud of every day.

Action is all-important. You can meditate on manifestations all day, but it takes action to make them happen.

Healers go through a process. First, we believe, then we know, then we do. It's a piece of cake.

Whenever possible, hurt no one and nothing.

See the truth in people, and still love them. You can love all people – including the mean ones – as long as you are connected to the Creator.

Each person is important. Each person is a spark of the Creator, and they should be valued as such. Take time to honor the God spark. I am constantly reminded how all of us are part of All That Is. Every heart is important.

You gotta laugh! A sense of humor is the best way to cope with the challenges that life has to offer. After all, life just is.

It just is.

Every experience matters. Every decision has brought you to this point in life. You can change, you can add to your self, you can redirect your self, but only *you* can decide who you are and what you can create and manifest. To know your self is to create your self. Ultimately, we create our own reality.

Only the dead fish go with the flow. You must go toward the truth even if it is up-river.

Not everyone is going to agree with you or like you. This is free agency, one of the most important Laws of the universe.

Live your life as if there are no secrets. Live as an open book, as if you could tell anyone what you did each day. Sometimes the best secrets are kept by sharing them with the world.

People say that time begins to accelerate the older you get, but I have never found this to be so. To me, time passes the same as when I was a child. What I have learned about the blessing of the passage of time is that no matter what obstacle is in your life, it will pass – everything changes with time. However, there are times when I wish that time would stand still just so I could enjoy the moment.

Remember, this is just a moment in time.

Wanna Play?

•••

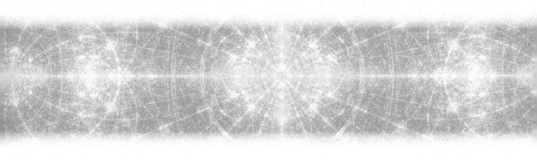

GLOSSARY

Belief system
An individual's or social group's set of beliefs about what is right and wrong and what is true and false. Beliefs that are stacked on top of one another make up the belief system or chain of beliefs.

Belief work
A process of pulling and replacing **belief system**s.

Conscious
Being fully aware of actions and self. It is theorized that the conscious mind only runs 10 percent of the brain and the **subconscious** the remaining 90 percent.

Core beliefs
See four levels of belief

Council of Twelve
Higher beings that can be called on for impartial advice, assistance, and judgment.

The Creator of All That Is
The most intelligent, perfect love energy in which everything in existence is created.

Digging work
A process to find a chain of beliefs that are stacked on top of one another and to change the bottom or key belief.

Divine timing
Knowing your destiny and allowing the universe to come in and help you.

Downloads
A process of witnessing positive affirmations coming down from the **Creator of All That Is** into the mind as though it were a computer.

Energy test
A process in Thetahealing to test for **belief systems**.

Four aspects

Each of the **four levels of belief** has four aspects: survival, undercurrent, ego self, and higher self and the soul.

Four levels of belief

There are four different levels of belief: core beliefs, genetic beliefs, history beliefs, and soul beliefs:

- **Core beliefs:** The first of the **four levels of belief**. Behavior patterns in the **subconscious** mind from this life – mostly stemming from childhood – which have become a part of our **programs**. Often, this is an effort on the part of the subconscious to protect us and keep us safe. When working on this level, the practitioner will witness changes in the frontal lobe.

- **Genetic beliefs:** The second of the **four levels of belief** we inherit genetic beliefs from our parents and ancestors, up to seven generations forward and seven generations back.

- **History beliefs:** The third of the **four levels of belief**. These beliefs are from past-life memories, and there are many reasons for them, including:

  - Behavior patterns from more than seven generations in the past.

  - Energies from the Akashic records.

- Collective consciousness memories from personal past-life experiences

The past-life energy of others left as imprints from past experiences imbedded in inanimate objects. In every grain of sand, there are memories of everything that has ever lived on the Earth – experiences that we carry into the present.

- **Soul beliefs:** The final of the **four levels of belief.** These are the deepest and most pervasive of all the belief programs. If a belief is repeated on more than one level, it can go all the way to the soul level. Even though your soul is from God, it is always learning.

Healing system
A process of co-creating using a Theta state to witness the **Creator of All That Is** doing a healing. Helping the body to heal and recover.

History beliefs
See four levels of belief

Programs
These are behavior patterns that have been created by beliefs in the mind.

Seven Planes of Existence

In ThetaHealing the term is used to describe the seven different realms that are separated by the movement of atoms:

- First Plane: Atoms come together, moving slowly to form solids, e.g., minerals

- Second Plane: Atoms begin to move faster to form plants

- Third Plane: Realm of animals and proteins

- Fourth Plane: Spirit realm

- Fifth Plane: Realm of the ascended masters

- Sixth Plane: The Laws of the universe

- Seventh Plane: The pure energy of creation, which folds into our universe and creates quarks, which create protons, neutrons, and electrons; which create atoms, which create molecules.

Sleep cycle

A time period of usually eight hours in which deep theta- and delta-states of sleep anchor new knowledge in the brain.

Soul beliefs

See four levels of belief

Subconscious

The part of the mind that runs the autonomic systems of the body, as well as some feelings and memories. Its main objective is to keep us safe and alive. The mental activity just below the threshold of consciousness.

Theta state

A very deep state of relaxation, a dream state at four to seven cycles per second. A creative, inspirational state characterized by spiritual sensations. *See also* **healing system**.

THETAHEALING®
SEMINARS AND
BOOKS

ThetaHealing is an energy-healing modality founded by Vianna Stibal, with certified instructors around the world. The seminars and books of ThetaHealing are designed as a therapeutic self-help guide to developing the ability of the mind to heal. ThetaHealing includes the following seminars and books:

ThetaHealing® seminars taught by certified ThetaHealing® Instructors

ThetaHealing Basic DNA 1 and 2 Practitioner Seminar

ThetaHealing Advanced DNA 2½ Practitioner Seminar

ThetaHealing Manifesting and Abundance Practitioner Seminar

ThetaHealing Intuitive Anatomy Practitioner Seminar

ThetaHealing Rainbow Children Practitioner Seminar

ThetaHealing Disease and Disorders Practitioner Seminar

ThetaHealing World Relations Practitioner Seminar

ThetaHealing DNA 3 Practitioner Seminar

ThetaHealing Animal Practitioner Seminar

ThetaHealing Dig Deeper Practitioner Seminar

ThetaHealing Plant Practitioner Seminar

ThetaHealing Soul Mate Practitioner Seminar

ThetaHealing Rhythm Practitioner Seminar

ThetaHealing Planes of Existence Practitioner Seminar

ThetaHealing Growing Your Relationship Instructor Classes

ThetaHealing You and Your Significant Other Seminar

ThetaHealing You and the Creator Seminar

ThetaHealing You and Your Inner Circle Seminar

ThetaHealing You and the Earth Seminar

ThetaHealing Planes of Existence 2 Seminar

Certification seminars taught exclusively by Vianna at the ThetaHealing® Institute of Knowledge

ThetaHealing Basic DNA Instructors' Seminar

ThetaHealing Advanced DNA 2½ Instructors' Seminar

ThetaHealing Manifesting and Abundance Instructors' Seminar

ThetaHealing Digging For Beliefs

ThetaHealing Intuitive Anatomy Instructors' Seminar

ThetaHealing Rainbow Children Instructors' Seminar

ThetaHealing Disease and Disorders Instructors' Seminar

ThetaHealing World Relations Instructors' Seminar

ThetaHealing DNA 3 Instructors' Seminar

ThetaHealing Animal Instructors' Seminar

ThetaHealing Dig Deeper Instructors' Seminar

ThetaHealing Plant Instructors' Seminar

ThetaHealing Soul Mate Instructors' Seminar

ThetaHealing Rhythm Instructors' Seminar

ThetaHealing Planes of Existence Instructors' Seminar

ThetaHealing Growing Your Relationship Certification Classes

ThetaHealing You and Your Significant Other Instructors' Seminar

ThetaHealing You and the Creator Instructors' Seminar

ThetaHealing You and Your Inner Circle Instructors' Seminar

ThetaHealing You and the Earth Instructors' Seminar

ThetaHealing Planes of Existence 2 Instructors' Seminar

ThetaHealing is always growing and expanding, and new courses are added often. Please visit www.ThetaHealing.com for latest updates.

Books

ThetaHealing® (Hay House, 2010, 2020)

Advanced ThetaHealing® (Hay House, 2011)

ThetaHealing® *Diseases and Disorders* (Hay House, 2011)

On the Wings of Prayer (Hay House, 2012)

ThetaHealing® *Rhythm for Finding Your Perfect Weight* (Hay House, 2013)

Seven Planes of Existence (Hay House, 2016)

ThetaHealing® *Digging for Beliefs* (Hay House) 2019

ABOUT THE AUTHOR

Vianna Stibal is the creator and founder of the spiritual philosophy, meditation, and healing technique known as ThetaHealing®. A renowned healer, author, and motivational speaker, Vianna conducts seminars with her husband, Guy, all over the world to people of all races, beliefs, and religions. As of 2019, she had trained thousands of instructors and an estimated 600,000 practitioners who are working in over 180 countries.

Vianna's technique takes the mind to a deep theta state (dream state) instantaneously. Using this state, she teaches her students to reestablish their conscious connection with the Creator of All That Is to facilitate spiritual, mental, emotional, and physical changes.

After witnessing her own healing, Vianna discovered how emotions and beliefs affect us on core, genetic, history, and soul levels. From this breakthrough, was born the belief work that became the heart and soul of ThetaHealing.

Belief work is a guide to find what we believe, why we believe, and how to change beliefs, change illness, understand the Creator's true plan, and create the reality we desire.

Vianna teaches that we are sparks of God creating our own reality, and that everything in our life serves a purpose. She is dedicated to sharing her love for the Creator of All That Is with an honest humor and a genuine kindness. Her trainings and books are life-changing and continue to help people all over the world.

www.thetahealing.com

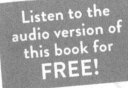

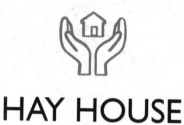

HAY HOUSE
Look within

Join the conversation about latest products, events, exclusive offers and more.

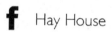 Hay House

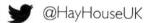 @HayHouseUK

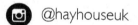 @hayhouseuk

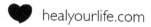 healyourlife.com

We'd love to hear from you!